T0206076

Data and Safety Monitoring Committees in Clinical Trials

Second Edition

Chapman & Hall/CRC Biostatistics Series

Editor-in-Chief

Shein-Chung Chow, Ph.D., Professor, Department of Biostatistics and Bioinformatics, Duke University School of Medicine, Durham, North Carolina

Series Editors

Byron Jones, Biometrical Fellow, Statistical Methodology, Integrated Information Sciences, Novartis Pharma AG, Basel, Switzerland

Jen-pei Liu, Professor, Division of Biometry, Department of Agronomy, National Taiwan University, Taipei, Taiwan

Karl E. Peace, Georgia Cancer Coalition, Distinguished Cancer Scholar, Senior Research Scientist and Professor of Biostatistics, Jiann-Ping Hsu College of Public Health, Georgia Southern University, Statesboro, Georgia

Bruce W. Turnbull, Professor, School of Operations Research and Industrial Engineering, Cornell University, Ithaca, New York

Published Titles

Adaptive Design Methods in Clinical Trials, Second Edition
Shein-Chung Chow and Mark Chang

Adaptive Designs for Sequential Treatment Allocation
Alessandro Baldi Antognini and Alessandra Giovagnoli

Adaptive Design Theory and Implementation Using SAS and R, Second Edition
Mark Chang

Advanced Bayesian Methods for Medical Test Accuracy
Lyle D. Broemeling

Analyzing Longitudinal Clinical Trial Data: A Practical Guide
Craig Mallinckrodt and Ilya Lipkovich

Applied Biclustering Methods for Big and High-Dimensional Data Using R
Adetayo Kasim, Ziv Shkedy, Sebastian Kaiser, Sepp Hochreiter, and Willem Talloen

Applied Meta-Analysis with R
Ding-Geng (Din) Chen and Karl E. Peace

Applied Surrogate Endpoint Evaluation Methods with SAS and R
Ariel Alonso, Theophile Bigirumurame, Tomasz Burzykowski, Marc Buyse, Geert Molenberghs, Leacky Muchene, Nolen Joy Perualila, Ziv Shkedy, and Wim Van der Elst

Basic Statistics and Pharmaceutical Statistical Applications, Second Edition
James E. De Muth

Bayesian Adaptive Methods for Clinical Trials
Scott M. Berry, Bradley P. Carlin, J. Jack Lee, and Peter Muller

Bayesian Analysis Made Simple: An Excel GUI for WinBUGS
Phil Woodward

Bayesian Designs for Phase I–II Clinical Trials
Ying Yuan, Hoang Q. Nguyen, and Peter F. Thall

Bayesian Methods for Measures of Agreement
Lyle D. Broemeling

Bayesian Methods for Repeated Measures
Lyle D. Broemeling

Bayesian Methods in Epidemiology
Lyle D. Broemeling

Bayesian Methods in Health Economics
Gianluca Baio

Bayesian Missing Data Problems: EM, Data Augmentation and Noniterative Computation
Ming T. Tan, Guo-Liang Tian, and Kai Wang Ng

Published Titles

Bayesian Modeling in Bioinformatics
Dipak K. Dey, Samiran Ghosh,
and Bani K. Mallick

Benefit-Risk Assessment in Pharmaceutical Research and Development
Andreas Sashegyi, James Felli,
and Rebecca Noel

Benefit-Risk Assessment Methods in Medical Product Development: Bridging Qualitative and Quantitative Assessments
Qi Jiang and Weili He

Bioequivalence and Statistics in Clinical Pharmacology, Second Edition
Scott Patterson and Byron Jones

Biosimilar Clinical Development: Scientific Considerations and New Methodologies
Kerry B. Barker, Sandeep M. Menon,
Ralph B. D'Agostino, Sr., Siyan Xu, and Bo Jin

Biosimilars: Design and Analysis of Follow-on Biologics
Shein-Chung Chow

Biostatistics: A Computing Approach
Stewart J. Anderson

Cancer Clinical Trials: Current and Controversial Issues in Design and Analysis
Stephen L. George, Xiaofei Wang,
and Herbert Pang

Causal Analysis in Biomedicine and Epidemiology: Based on Minimal Sufficient Causation
Mikel Aickin

Clinical and Statistical Considerations in Personalized Medicine
Claudio Carini, Sandeep Menon, and Mark Chang

Clinical Trial Data Analysis using R
Ding-Geng (Din) Chen and Karl E. Peace

Clinical Trial Methodology
Karl E. Peace and Ding-Geng (Din) Chen

Computational Methods in Biomedical Research
Ravindra Khattree and Dayanand N. Naik

Computational Pharmacokinetics
Anders Källén

Confidence Intervals for Proportions and Related Measures of Effect Size
Robert G. Newcombe

Controversial Statistical Issues in Clinical Trials
Shein-Chung Chow

Data Analysis with Competing Risks and Intermediate States
Ronald B. Geskus

Data and Safety Monitoring Committees in Clinical Trials, Second Edition
Jay Herson

Design and Analysis of Animal Studies in Pharmaceutical Development
Shein-Chung Chow and Jen-pei Liu

Design and Analysis of Bioavailability and Bioequivalence Studies, Third Edition
Shein-Chung Chow and Jen-pei Liu

Design and Analysis of Bridging Studies
Jen-pei Liu, Shein-Chung Chow,
and Chin-Fu Hsiao

Design & Analysis of Clinical Trials for Economic Evaluation & Reimbursement: An Applied Approach Using SAS & STATA
Iftekhar Khan

Design and Analysis of Clinical Trials for Predictive Medicine
Shigeyuki Matsui, Marc Buyse,
and Richard Simon

Design and Analysis of Clinical Trials with Time-to-Event Endpoints
Karl E. Peace

Design and Analysis of Non-Inferiority Trials
Mark D. Rothmann, Brian L. Wiens,
and Ivan S. F. Chan

Difference Equations with Public Health Applications
Lemuel A. Moyé and Asha Seth Kapadia

DNA Methylation Microarrays: Experimental Design and Statistical Analysis
Sun-Chong Wang and Arturas Petronis

Published Titles

Chapman & Hall/CRC Biostatistics Series

Data and Safety Monitoring Committees in Clinical Trials

Second Edition

Jay Herson

Johns Hopkins Bloomberg School of Public Health

Baltimore, Maryland, USA

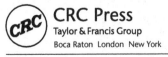

CRC Press
Taylor & Francis Group
Boca Raton London New York

CRC Press is an imprint of the
Taylor & Francis Group, an **informa** business
A CHAPMAN & HALL BOOK

CRC Press
Taylor & Francis Group
6000 Broken Sound Parkway NW, Suite 300
Boca Raton, FL 33487-2742

First issued in paperback 2019

ISBN-13: 978-1-4987-8410-8 (hbk)
ISBN-13: 978-0-367-26127-6 (pbk)

Library of Congress Cataloging-in-Publication Data

Names: Herson, Jay, author.
Title: Data and safety monitoring committees in clinical trials / Jay Herson, Ph.D.
Description: Second edition. | Boca Raton : Taylor & Francis, 2017. | Series: Chapman & Hall/CRC biostatistics series | Includes bibliographical references and index.
Identifiers: LCCN 2016026387 | ISBN 9781498784108 (hardback)
Subjects: LCSH: Drugs--Testing--Evaluation. | Drugs--Testing--Statistical methods--Evaluation.
Classification: LCC RM301.27 .H47 2017 | DDC 615.1/9--dc23
LC record available at https://lccn.loc.gov/2016026387

Visit the Taylor & Francis Web site at
http://www.taylorandfrancis.com

and the CRC Press Web site at
http://www.crcpress.com

To the patients who volunteer for clinical trials—past, present, and future.

Contents

Preface to the First Edition

This is a book about *best practices* in safety monitoring through data monitoring committees (DMC) in pharmaceutical industry clinical trials. It will be useful for those who have served on DMCs and are interested in what was done well and what could have been done better and those contemplating serving on their first committee.

I can still remember that winter morning 20 years ago in San Antonio, when Frank Rockhold asked me at a biostatistical meeting we were attending if I could organize a DMC for a gastrointestinal drug his company was developing. Frank, his talented colleagues, and I worked out a plan and the first DMC in pharmaceutical industry trials was born. At the time, I headed a contract research organization (CRO) in Houston known as Applied Logic Associates (ALA). Since then, that company has provided statistical support to more than 50 DMCs and I have served as statistical member on DMCs for about 30 additional trials. The art and science of safety monitoring through DMCs has reached adolescence and it is time to review, and perhaps debate, best practices. There can be no better time than now, when regulatory agencies worldwide are facing considerable challenges in drug safety for both premarket and postmarketed drugs.

In the world of drug development, clinical issues and statistical issues cannot be separated. All issues are scientific. All use *applied logic*. This is the approach to this book. It is written in the style of my *Herson's Handout* column that appeared in the ALA newsletter *Under the Curve*, 1991–2004. This was a style appropriate for all drug development professionals regardless of degrees held. The book assumes that the reader has a basic knowledge of clinical trials, clinical operations, and good clinical practices.

Chapter 1 is introductory. It points out the differences between clinical trials sponsored by the federal government and those sponsored by pharmaceutical firms. These differences explain why DMCs operate a little differently for private sector–sponsored trials. We learn that pharmaceutical companies themselves differ by their size and the terms Big Pharma, Middle Pharma, and Infant Pharma are defined. Another important definition is that of stewardship. If there had to be one word to define the role of DMCs it would be stewardship. We also learn the limitations for uncovering safety issues in a single premarket clinical program and provide a rule of thumb for assessing the sensitivity of a clinical program to uncovering adverse events.

Chapter 2 details the organization of safety monitoring describing the interactions of the sponsor, the DMC, the Data Analysis Center (DAC), the Institutional Review Board (IRB), and the regulatory agencies. Tables in the chapter offer checklists of desirable characteristics of a sponsor representative, a DAC organization, questions to ask oneself, and the sponsor before agreeing to join a DMC.

Chapter 3 explains the nature of DMC meetings. Of special importance is the orientation meeting. In this section, the items usually included in the DMC Charter are listed. From this, the extent of DMC responsibilities for the trial, reporting procedures, serious adverse event data flow, masking (blinding) policy, and many other important agreements that must be made between the sponsor, DAC, and DMC at the outset of the trial are detailed in the text and tables. Another table presents a sample agenda format for DMC meetings that has proven more useful than a mere list of topics to be discussed.

Chapter 4 is an introduction to clinical issues. Here, we will see how the safety data reviewed by DMCs arise. We learn the important distinction between adverse events, serious adverse events, and severity of adverse events. The current state of the art of adverse event coding is described. The impact of multinational trials and the cultural, political, and medical practice issues relevant to DMC operations are described.

In Chapter 5, we investigate statistical methods useful for DMCs. It is emphasized that statistical significance of a treatment difference for a safety parameter is neither a necessary nor sufficient reason to terminate a trial. We see some useful graphical and tabular data displays and review statistical methods for testing hypotheses and creating confidence intervals for various measures of treatment differences in safety. The methods are illustrated with data from an actual clinical trial. Every DMC faces problems of multiplicity and this concept is explained and use of the false discovery rate is presented as a means of controlling multiplicity. The chapter includes an introduction to likelihood methods for assessing evidence. Much of the work in this area has been done by my graduate school advisor, Professor Richard Royall. I have found the methods useful for DMC work. I am excited to be able to present the methods here. The chapter closes with a brief description of the role of Bayesian methods for safety analysis. A table is presented summarizing all methods discussed in the chapter along with their advantages and disadvantages for DMC use.

Chapter 6 continues in the inference vein with a description of the biases and pitfalls in analyzing safety data. Sources of bias arise from unmasking, incomplete follow-up, spontaneous versus solicited adverse event data collection, early termination due to efficacy, and the problems introduced by slicing and dicing the adverse event descriptions into many subgroups within a body system (granularity). Finally, the concept of competing risks in adverse event incidence is presented, particularly in the case where there is differential follow-up between treatment groups due to a treatment effect in a primary efficacy endpoint.

We now arrive at Chapter 7, where we apply our knowledge from prior chapters to data monitoring committee decisions. We review the types of decisions that DMCs can make as well as the environment in which they are made. We see the steps that can be taken when a safety issue arises and the potential pitfalls in incorporating data from past clinical trials into the decision-making process.

Chapter 8 might also be called an epilogue. It deals with emerging issues in drug development that affect DMC operations. The issues are divided into those that arise from advances in technology and those that arise through the maturation of the DMC process. In the former, we take up adaptive designs. Of particular importance is the situation when an adaptive change is taking place on the basis of efficacy but, due to safety, the DMC feels that this change will not be in the interest of patient safety. Other technology changes are the advent of real-time SAE reporting and the potential of certain adverse events to be biomarkers for efficacy. In the area of maturation of DMC processes, training of DMC members, CROs, DACs, and even sponsor representatives to the DMC paradigm is very important and how can we create the supply of qualified individuals to meet the demands. Sponsors have encountered problems with cost control as DMCs ask for more data than was originally planned. Suggestions are given for dealing with this situation. What happens when pharmaceutical companies merge or out-license the product the DMC is deliberating? How do we ensure that independent review of patient safety will continue? New medical journal policies requiring DMCs and independent statistical review will also affect DMC operations and are covered here as well.

At the end of each chapter, the reader will find a Q & A section called DMCounselor. The questions provide a behind-the-scenes glimpse of DMC meetings, interactions with sponsors, multinational issues, personality conflicts, and especially the problems that Infant Pharma faces in providing independent review in the same manner as Big Pharma. All cases raised in this section are real. They were either my own personal experience or those of others. All details of the cases have been changed for confidentiality but the conundrums remain. Some readers may not agree with the solutions that I provide in my answer but at least they can see issues they may not have thought of before.

A glossary is presented giving definitions of most of the technical terms used in the text and the appendix contains a table of adverse events reported for selected marketed drugs in placebo-controlled trials. It is referred to at various points in the text to illustrate safety concepts.

I explain in the text that I use the term *sponsor* where others might use *company*. I use the term *patient* as the clinical unit in our trials. I realize that in some indications *subject* would be more appropriate but I chose patient for consistency. I use the term *drug* as a synonym for *intervention*. The latter term would include biologics and medical devices. I felt that most readers are used to this terminology. Indeed, the Food and Drug Administration and the Drug Information Association deal with interventions broader than just drugs.

About a year after completing my first statistics course as an undergraduate, I noticed that the professor had published his own textbook on the subject. When I asked him how long it took him to write the book, he replied "Well it is hard to say, I have been teaching for twenty years." I now understand what he meant. Although writing this book may have taken 1 year it represents

20 years of experience. This also means that it will be impossible for me to thank all those people who I have learned from. I certainly must thank Frank Rockhold for introducing me to the DMC concept. The many employees of ALA, too numerous to name here, for their insight into the details, such as MedDRA and related software, their development of efficient methodology, and the realization that protecting patient safety was just as important as hitting a home run in efficacy. During my years as president of ALA, I became intimately aware of the issues facing Infant Pharma and am grateful for the opportunity to present them here. There have been many DMCs. If I had to single out one DMC experience it would be the one that lasted longest. My hat goes off to ophthalmologists Alan Bird, Don D'Amico and Ron Klein, DAC biostatistician Emmanuel Quinaux, and sponsor representative Harvey Masonson for all they taught me while we had the privilege of working on the first vascular endothelial growth factor used in ophthalmology. It was a very educational 6 years.

I am so grateful for the Biostatistics Department at the Johns Hopkins Bloomberg School of Public Health in Baltimore for welcoming me into the department after my semiretirement and offering me the physical and intellectual environment conducive to writing a book. Among the Johns Hopkins family, Scott Zeger brought me into the department in 2004 and Richard Royall not only introduced me to likelihood methods when I was his student but set the example for me by writing such a fine book on the subject. Jeff Blume and Elizabeth Garrett-Mayer also shared a lot of ideas about likelihood and were a help with the graphs.

I thank biostatisticians Dennis Dixon, Janet Wittes, and Marc Buyse not only for our long friendship but also for teaching me the differences between government and private industry trials. I thank Janet also for her official responsibility of reviewing this manuscript and making so many important suggestions and corrections.

This book would never have come about if David Grubbs of the Taylor & Francis Group had not approached me about writing a book and offering me encouragement along the way. Taylor & Francis could not have provided me with a better project coordinator than Marsha Pronin.

Last, but certainly not least, I must thank my wife Linda for enduring my writing obsession and providing so much encouragement for what is the equivalent of a second doctoral dissertation some 37 years after the first. Yes Linda, I'll clean up the room now.

I hope that the many drug development professionals who read this book will find it useful in starting a dialog on best practices beyond the point of just writing a charter and scheduling meetings. I hope that those talented readers who have not yet served on a DMC will consider doing so. It is an important and rewarding experience.

Jay Herson, PhD
July 15, 2008

Preface to the Second Edition

When the first edition of this book was published in 2009, a second edition was the furthest thing from my mind. However, in the past 2 years alone, we have seen a huge impetus of regulations and books on safety in drug development. The big push is to guide safety monitoring and analysis toward risk (adverse events) versus benefit (efficacy) and to reduce the paperwork in expedited reporting of adverse events. Terms such as SUSARs, SMQs, PSAP, companion diagnostics, safety assessment committees, and so forth, did not exist, at least in my vocabulary, when I created the first edition in 2008.

The new regulations have been complemented by the development of new statistical methods, which are also described here so that DMC members will have a reference if they should appear at a meeting. Meta-analysis, use of outside data, Bayesian methods, and causal inference are more common today than they were in 2008, so I have given them more ink.

The first edition mentioned the efficacy analysis responsibilities of DMCs but gave no details. This edition provides the statistical elements of planned interim analysis with group sequential methods, conditional power, futility, and so on.

I have introduced some new ideas of my own. While I applaud the SPERT recommendation of the PSAP (Program Safety Analysis Plan), I see much of that as a sponsor guide toward a final safety analysis. Thus, I have introduced the notion of a Data Review Plan (DRP), which would be solely for DMC use. For those who have been concerned about DMC independence from the sponsor, I introduce the ideas of the DMC members being appointed jointly by sponsor and regulators but compensated by regulators. We have seen more than a few cases of data fraud in clinical trials and we expect more cases to come up in the future with the advent of centralized statistical monitoring. Thus, I have added my idea of a Fraud Recovery Plan, which could be used to salvage a clinical trial when some cases of data fraud are found. These items have been added with the objective of beginning what I think would be useful discussions of these issues, something like a draft guidance issued by a regulatory agency.

I have participated in many more DMCs since the first edition and have greatly expanded the popular DMCounseler Q & A at the end of every chapter with new scenarios representing my recent experiences and those of others. As with the first edition, the details of the clinical trials have been changed to protect the innocent.

At the end of Chapters 3 through 8, I have added tables to indicate useful DRP items and potential DMC responsibilities implied in that chapter. I have aggregated these chapter tables in Appendix Table A.2 for the DRP and Table A.3 for the DMC. I hope these will be useful to sponsors and DMC members in preparing DRPs and DMC Charters.

Once again, I must thank David Grubbs and his talented colleagues at Chapman & Hall/CRC Press for encouraging me to write the second edition and for all of the support along the way. My hat also goes off to the many people who have written books on statistical methods for drug safety over the past few years. I have referenced so many of their chapters. I must paraphrase a much-quoted Groucho Marx phrase "I would never serve on a committee that would have me as a member." I do not like committee work but stand in awe of those who toil on industry panels such as SPERT, BRAT, and PRISMA all of which are spelled out in this edition. Their work has really moved the field forward. Our colleagues in the regulatory agencies have put much thought into the new drug safety guidelines and it has been my pleasure to relate their words to DMC responsibilities.

My association with the Biostatistics Department at the Johns Hopkins Bloomberg School of Public Health continues to be rewarding and to provide the stimulating environment for this undertaking and for the many ideas I get from faculty and present and former students.

Again, I thank my wife, Linda, for putting up with my obsession with still another book. Fortunately it did not prevent us from doing the travel we enjoy so much.

Like the first edition, the second edition is about best practices. I hope this book will help those of us who work on drug development and understand how best practices have evolved.

Jay Herson, PhD

List of Abbreviations

AE	adverse event
AESI	adverse event of special interest
ALA	Applied Logic Associates
APD	aggregate patient data
APPROVe	Adenomatous Polyp Prevention on Vioxx
AUC	area under the curve
BRAT	Benefit Risk Action Team
CDC	Centers for Disease Control and Prevention
CHW	Chi Hung Wang method of sample size reestimation
CI	confidence interval
CIOMS	Council of International Organizations of Medical Sciences
CRA	clinical research associate
CRF	case report form
CRO	contract research organization
CTCAE	Common Terminology Criteria for Adverse Events
DAC	Data Analysis Center
DFDR	double false discovery rate
DFS	disease-free survival
DRP	Data Review Plan
DTS	dynamic treatment strategy
DMC	Data Monitoring Committee
EMA	European Medicines Agency
ETASU	Elements to Assure Safe Use
FDA	Food and Drug Administration
FDR	false discovery rate
FRP	fraud recovery plan
FWER	family-wise error rate
HDL	high-density lipoprotein
HIV	human immunodeficiency virus
ICH	International Collaboration on Harmonisation
IFPMA	International Federation of Pharmaceutical Manufacturers and Associations
IPD	individual patient data
IQWiG	German Institute for Quality and Efficiency in Health Care
IRB	Institutional Review Board
ISRC	Internal Safety Review Committee
ISS	integrated summary of safety
ITE	insufficient therapeutic effect
LDL	low-density lipoprotein
LR	likelihood ratio

LRC	lipids research clinics
MD	doctor of medicine
MACE	major adverse cardiac event
MedDRA	*Medical Dictionary for Regulatory Activities*
MOOC	massive online open course
MSSO	Maintenance Support and Service Organization
NCI	National Cancer Institute
NIAID	National Institute of Allergic and Infectious Disease
NICE	National Institute of Health and Clinical Excellence
NIH	National Institutes of Health
NNH	number needed to harm
NNT	number needed to treat
NSAID	nonsteroidal anti-inflammatory drug
OS	overall survival
PAC	pulmonary arterial catheter
PDUFA	Prescription Drug User Fee Act
PFS	progression-free survival
PharmD	doctor of pharmacy
PhD	doctor of philosophy
PRISMA	Preferred Reporting Items for Systematic Reviews and Meta-Analysis
PRO-CTCAE	patient-reported outcome version of CTCAE
PSAP	Program Safety Analysis Plan
R&D	research and development
RB	risk–benefit
REMS	risk evaluation and mitigation strategy
SAC	Safety Assessment Committee
SAE	serious adverse event
SAP	statistical analysis plan
SC	Steering Committee
SE	standard error
SMART	sequential multiple assignment randomized trial
SMP	safety monitoring plan
SMQ	standardized MedDRA query
SOC	system organ class
SOP	standard operating procedure
SPERT	Safety Planning, Evaluation, and Reporting Team
SUSAR	Serious Unexpected Suspected Adverse Reaction
UK	United Kingdom
U.S.	United States
VA	Veterans Administration
WHO	World Health Organization

1

Introduction

PREVIEW   The data monitoring committee is the keystone of the steward-ship and the scientific/ethical integrity of a clinical trial. The independent review of safety in clinical trials began in the public-funded clinical trials and has become the mainstream in pharmaceutical industry clinical trials today. After acknowledging the limitations of a single clinical trial to find rare adverse events, a rule of thumb for measuring the sensitivity of a clinical program that observes adverse events of various frequencies is presented. Issues involved in safety monitoring may differ between the size of industry sponsor and public versus private company.

KEY WORDS: *adverse event, Big Pharma, confirmatory clinical trial, data moni-toring committee, Infant Pharma, masked, Middle Pharma, serious adverse event, sponsor*

1.1 What Is a Data Monitoring Committee (DMC)?

Professor Jerome Cornfield once defined a clinical trial as *cogent* description (Cornfield 1973). It has become clear that objectivity in reviewing accumulat-ing data in clinical trials is extremely important in maintaining cogency. One factor that can operate against cogency is *bias*. We will discuss the concept of bias in Chapter 6, but for now, let's define it as a conscious or unconscious lack of objectivity due to a sponsor staff's interest in getting the experimental treatment approved by regulatory agencies. Clinical trial sponsor staff can introduce bias into trial conduct if they review efficacy data during the trial and may have a tendency to underplay the importance of adverse events that present during the trial. This is especially true in oncology trials which are usually conducted with sponsor staff, investigators, and patients all aware of treatment assignment. Although sponsors tended to claim that their trial management did not introduce bias, the current feeling is that if clinical trial results are to be persuasive to regulatory agencies, practicing physicians, and the general public, even the appearance of bias must be avoided. The prob-lem is complicated by the fact that investigators and others associated with the trial can also introduce bias. While bias reduction is important for scien-tific and regulatory reasons, it has also become evident that objective review of accumulating data is necessary to protect patient safety.

In the late 1980s, following the example of clinical trials run by the U.S. federal government through agencies such as the National Institutes of Health (NIH), the Veterans Administration (VA) and the Centers for Disease Control and Prevention (CDC), the British Medical Research Council, and the French INSERM, the pharmaceutical industry began to form DMCs. These committees took on various names and were of various forms. Initially some of these committees included members who were sponsor staff but regulatory agencies took a dim view of this practice. Eventually, membership evolved to individuals who were not members of the sponsor staff but were physicians of appropriate specialties and experienced clinical trial biostatisticians who could be trusted to review efficacy and safety data in such a way that bias is minimized. In subsequent chapters, we will review "best practices" for minimizing bias and for DMC operations in general. This book will concentrate on the safety role of the DMC in industry-sponsored trials. Safety data constitute 85% of data collected in clinical trials submitted to the U.S. Food and Drug Administration (Rochester 2008), are evaluated more subjectively than efficacy data, and, experience shows, constitute about 90% of DMC operations.

A recent draft guidance by the FDA on safety assessment practices introduces the term "Safety Assessment Committee (SAC)." The role of this committee is broader than that of the DMC. While the DMC will consist entirely outside consultants, the SAC will consist of sponsor internal as well as outside experts and will integrate safety information from a development program with information from other clinical trials of the same or similar drugs, preclinical studies, epidemiologic studies, and so on, in order to form a complete impression on emerging adverse events. There is also considerable overlap between DMC and SAC responsibilities and there may be some common members to both committees. There is no reason that a DMC cannot be a subcommittee of an SAC. Until there is some experience with the SAC concept, there is likely to be confusion as to who has the last word on the experimental drug's safety profile. For now, it is important to note that the DMC is smaller and more focused than the SAC. We will continue to refer to the key safety committee as the DMC but, going forward, the reader should expect to see the term *safety assessment committee* appear in the literature (U.S. Food and Drug Administration 2015a).

1.2 Some Definitions

It will be useful to provide some brief definitions of important terms. We will return to these terms to provide more rigorous definitions later in the book.

The *sponsor* of a trial is the organization that has the ultimate responsibility for reporting the results to the regulatory authorities. For our purposes, it will most often be a pharmaceutical or biotechnology company but it could be a university, government agency, or, in the case of orphan drugs, a patient–parent support group.

An *adverse event* (AE) is any unfavorable and unintended sign (e.g., including an abnormal laboratory finding), symptom, or disease temporally associated with the use of a drug, whether or not considered related to the drug. An adverse event is deemed *treatment-emergent* if the adverse event is not a manifestation of a condition that existed prior to the clinical trial. It is not always easy to make this distinction. A *serious* adverse event (SAE) is any untoward medical occurrence that, at any dose, results in death, is life-threatening, requires inpatient hospitalization, or prolongation of existing hospitalization. This is the regulatory definition. We will see in Chapter 4, that this definition may generate different types of adverse events as serious in different countries due to differences in hospitalization policy.

The reader will be familiar with patients and possibly investigators being *blinded* to treatment assignment. In deference to our ophthalmology colleagues, we will use the term *masked* as a synonym for blinded. When treatment assignment is not masked to anyone we usually use the term *open label.*

The term *monitoring* is used in several different contexts in the pharmaceutical industry. *Statistical monitoring* refers to making calculations on accumulating efficacy data to justify early termination of a clinical trial (Proschan, Lan, and Wittes 2006) and/or sample size reestimation (Chuang-Stein, Anderson, Gallo et al. 2006). *Safety monitoring* by sponsor staff and DMC members refers to continual review of accumulating safety data during the trial. *Site monitoring* is a quality control procedure applied periodically during the trial by sponsor or contract clinical research associates (CRAs) (Woodin and Schneider 2003). In Chapter 8, we will review the newly emerging science of centralized statistical monitoring.

1.3 DMC in Federal Government–Sponsored Clinical Trials versus Pharmaceutical Industry Clinical Trials

DMCs had long been included in federal government–sponsored clinical trials before they appeared in pharmaceutical industry clinical trials. The latter took on a different form from the former due to differences in the characteristics of the trials being conducted (Herson 1993). Table 1.1 provides a summary of differences between federal government–sponsored trials and private industry sponsored trials. The federal government trials that are primarily *research or science* oriented with a public audience are sometimes community based (see, e.g., Djunaedi, Sommer, Pandji et al. 1988) and most often involve drugs already approved such as the Women's Health Initiative progestin trial (Writing Group for the Women's Health Initiative Investigators 2002; Wittes, Barrett-Connor, Braunwald et al. 2007). Industry

TABLE 1.1

Characteristics of Clinical Trials Utilizing DMCs by Sponsorship

Characteristics	Federal Government Sponsored	Private Industry Sponsored
Purpose	Advance medical research	Product approval
Activity	Research	Development
Orientation	Science	Product
Sampling unit	Community or patient	Patient
Audience	Public	Regulatory agency
At design stage	Know the question	"Know" the answer
Approval status of study drugs	Often approved drugs	Premarket, experimental
Design and analysis methods	Freedom to be creative	Must adhere to regulatory agency requirements
Pace	Careful, deliberate	Aggressive
Data quality control	Each trial can establish its own standards	Must adhere to high standards of good clinical practices
Financing	Federal budget or grants to universities	Corporate
Potential for conflict of interest	Lower than private industry sponsored	Higher than federal government sponsored
Type of trial	One trial, large number of patients, and long duration	Several trials with small number of patients and short follow-up time

trials are patient based and *development or product* oriented with the goal of convincing regulatory agencies that a new product should be approved and then reaching a market segment of patients through physicians. To illustrate this distinction consider the NIH-sponsored Lipids Research Clinics (LRC) trials (Lipids Research Clinics Program 1984a,b). At the LRC, design stage researchers asked the question "Does cholestyramine treatment to lower low density lipoprotein (LDL) for patients with hyperlipidemia have an effect on mortality and morbidity?" After 10 years of *research*, a positive result was found. Then, private industry was able to follow with *development* trials of fewer patients and shorter duration to show that lovastatin, for example, was effective in lowering LDL (Havel, Hunninghake, Illingworth et al. 1987). This conclusion was considered acceptable for approval since the NIH trial had established that lowering LDL had a positive effect on a clinically significant endpoint. When this pivotal trial began, the sponsor research staff "knew" the answer, that is, on the basis of the preliminary trials, they had confidence that the construct they designed would result in a positive outcome.

DMCs in NIH-sponsored trials are usually involved in trial design, sample size requirements, data analysis methods, data quality, publications policy, investigator evaluation, and so on, in addition to efficacy and safety review. These responsibilities become more complicated when, in addition to DMCs, the NIH trials include *steering committees* and *endpoint adjudication committees*.

The duties of DMCs operating within private industry trials are narrower in scope. However, some industry-sponsored trials also have these two types of committees. The roles of these committees will be described further in Chapter 2.

Lachin (2004) has indicated that there is more of a chance for conflict of interest in private industry trials than in government-sponsored trials. Pharmaceutical firms have learned that good science and objectivity are the best strategies for shortening the time to approval. Thus, DMCs in the pharmaceutical industry evolved as "blue ribbon" panels for independent certification on issues such as adjudication of efficacy endpoints, conduct of planned interim analyses, and safety monitoring. DMCs in the pharmaceutical industry are a node in an aggressive drug development process leading to marketing. There are considerable financial consequences in the outcome of the trial and numerous opportunities for bias and/or conflict of interest.

1.4 Stewardship

While sponsors retain DMCs to add to the objectivity and credibility of trials, DMC members can best fulfill their obligations to sponsors and patients by considering themselves responsible for the *stewardship* of the trial. This implies both the preservation of credibility of the trial and the aegis of patient safety. How this stewardship can best be carried out will be covered in later chapters of this book. For now, it is sufficient to note that DMC members must be proactive and consider themselves "board of directors" of the trial if they are to fulfill their responsibilities to the patients and sponsor.

1.5 Some Recent History

1.5.1 Development of DMCs in the Pharmaceutical Industry

One of the first-known DMCs in pharmaceutical industry clinical trials was the cimetidine stress ulcer clinical trial in 1988–1989 (Herson, Ognibene, Peura et al. 1992). This trial was conducted in intensive care units and was designed to compare cimetidine to placebo for prophylaxis of upper gastrointestinal bleeding due to stress (Martin, Booth, Karlstadt et al. 1993). The primary efficacy endpoint for this trial was prophylactic failure defined as the appearance of bright red blood and other bleeding-related outcomes. A supplementary definition of failure was "insufficient therapeutic effect" (ITE) which investigators could invoke at their discretion to remove a patient from the study if they feared the patient might begin to bleed. The sponsor

decided to create a DMC for independent and masked certification of bleeding data and determination if ITE decisions were made according to usual
clinical practice and safety monitoring including judgments on whether or
not death was disease related. The decision to involve a DMC in this trial
came from the sponsor's experience on earlier clinical trials for this product
where the possibility of bias in sponsor staff efficacy classifications raised
credibility issues with FDA. The sponsor and consultants used some aspects
of DMCs on NIH-sponsored trials to write the charter for their DMC.

Physicians chosen for this committee had expertise in gastrointestinal disease and emergency medicine. The data for DMC review were sent by the
sponsor to a contract research organization (CRO) with treatment assignments coming from a manufacturing office of the sponsor rather than from
those sponsor staff involved in the trial. All data processing for the DMC
was performed by the CRO. When the trial ended the DMC presented the
results to the sponsor. However, those sponsor staff members still evaluating
safety were not informed of results to avoid introduction of bias in ongoing
safety evaluations.

1.5.2 Guidance Documents: FDA, NIH, and ICH

Since DMCs first appeared in pharmaceutical trials in the early 1990s,
much has been written about the role of DMCs. Examples include the FDA
guidance finalized in 2006 (U.S. Food and Drug Administration 2006),
the International Conference on Harmonisation (ICH) E-3 guideline on
clinical study reports (International Conference on Harmonisation 1995),
the E-6 guideline on good clinical practices (International Conference
on Harmonisation 1996), and the E-9 guideline on statistical principles
(International Conference on Harmonisation 1998). The E2A guideline on clinical data safety management (International Conference on
Harmonisation 1994) provides some useful definitions but the vocabulary
and expedited reporting requirements have been superseded by some
recent FDA guidances to industry all of which have implications for DMC
responsibilities. In addition to the safety assessment guidance referred to
above, these would include the guidance on safety-reporting requirements
(U.S. Food and Drug Administration 2012), a risk-based approach to monitoring (U.S. Food and Drug Administration 2013), and risk evaluation and
mitigation strategies (U.S. Food and Drug Administration 2015b). We will
return to these guidances in later chapters.

Hemmings and Day (2004) provide a good discussion of regulatory issues
related to DMCs. Literature oriented toward NIH-sponsored trials would
include the NIH guidelines (U.S. National Institutes of Health 1998, 1999,
2000), the DAMOCLES literature search (Sydes, Spiegelhalter, Altman et al.
2004), and books by Ellenberg, Fleming, and DeMets (2002) and DeMets,
Furberg, and Friedman (2006). Recently some prestigious medical journals have adopted a policy of not publishing results of industry-sponsored

Phase III trials unless an independent DMC was involved (Fontanarosa, Flanagin, and DeAngelis 2005).

1.5.3 Other Vehicles for Patient Protection

DMCs are not the only source of protection of patient safety. Each clinical trial site (hospital, clinic, and doctor's office) comes under the auspices of an Institutional Review Board (IRB) or Ethics Committee which reviews protocols and their amendments and receives periodic safety reports. Each sponsor has internal safety review mechanisms and some larger medical institutions have internal DMC-like committees who review safety on ongoing trials regardless of sponsorship. The relationship between these entities and DMCs will be covered later in this book.

1.6 A DMC's Place in the Drug Development Cycle

1.6.1 Phases of Drug Development

Drug development is often broken into several phases—molecular, preclinical, exploratory, confirmatory, and postmarket (Scheiner 1997). The exploratory and confirmatory phases include those clinical trials that will be used for drug approval. The exploratory trials are often referred to as phase I and II. These trials are primarily *proof of concept* trials which establish dosage (maximum tolerated dose) and efficacy (minimum effective dose). Some prefer to call these trials *test of concept* rather than *proof* but in any case it is important to consider these early trials as *learning trials*. These are followed by the confirmatory trial(s) known as phase III. Here, we apply what we learned in earlier phases regarding dose, schedule, and appropriate patient populations to design a trial that is expected to demonstrate efficacy and safety with statistical precision. Phase III trials are sometimes called *pivotal* trials because they are the trials that will form the basis of the regulatory decision. The terms *confirmatory, phase III*, and *pivotal* will be used synonymously in this book.

1.6.2 Limitations of a Clinical Program for Revealing Safety Issues

The clinical program is conducted to produce evidence of efficacy and safety sufficient for marketing approval by regulatory agencies. This program will provide evidence of serious adverse events that occur with highest frequency. It must be understood that it is the DMC's role to consider these adverse events but, obviously, not to be responsible for all SAEs that may ever be associated with the drug during its lifetime.

TABLE 1.2

Clinical Trials Terminated Due to Safety

Drug	Indication in Trial	Risk	Trial Terminated
Torcetrapib	Raise HDL (high-density lipoprotein)	Increase in cardiovascular events and death	2006
Estrogen + progestin	Prevention of chronic disease	Invasive breast cancer, coronary heart disease	2002
Tirilazad	Head trauma	Death	1994
Rofecoxib	Polyp prevention	Thrombotic events	2004
Celecoxib	Polyp prevention	Thrombotic events	2004
Naproxen	Alzheimer's	Fear of thrombotic events	2004

A single pivotal clinical trial designed to demonstrate efficacy will not be able to assess rare events or those that represent delayed effects. The DMC may not gain an understanding of which AEs will become chronic during the duration of a clinical trial. Despite the limitations, several clinical trials have been terminated for safety in recent years. A partial listing is found in Table 1.2. In the period 2008–2010, 19% of phase II trials were terminated due to safety (17 of 87) and 21% of 83 products failed due to safety in phase III or during regulatory review (Arrowsmith 2011a,b).

In a clinical program, it is always useful to keep in mind the "rule of 3000/n" where n = the number of patients exposed to the drug in a clinical program. This calculation yields a lower bound on the sensitivity of the trial to detect adverse events on an incidence/1000 basis. For example if n = 1000 patients, then, the clinical program is likely to find at least one case of AEs that occurs at an incidence of 3000/1000 (= 3) or 3/1000. If n = 500, then, the clinical program would be sensitive to find at least one case that occurred with incidence 6/1000. To be able to find an adverse event that occurs at the rate of 1/100,000 a program of 300,000 patients would be required. This type of AE could only be found in postmarket surveillance. Table 1.3 presents a table for sensitivity for AE detection in a hypothetical clinical program for development of a diabetes drug. We

TABLE 1.3

Sensitivity to AE Detection in a Clinical Program for Development of a Diabetes Drug

Protocol No.	Description	n for This Protocol	AE Detection Rate/1000	n (Cumulative)	Cumulative AE Detection Rate/1000
11	26 weeks + 3 months extension	348	8.6	348	8.6
12	26 weeks + 3 months extension	406	7.4	754	4.0
21	26 weeks + 6 months extension	510	5.9	1264	2.4
22	26 weeks + 6 months extension	928	3.2	2192	1.4
31	52 weeks	604	5.0	2796	1.1

see that the sensitivity of the individual protocols to detect AEs ranges from 3.2 to 8.6/1000. As the program progresses, sensitivity does not drop below 3/1000 until the first 26-week + 6-month extension trial (protocol 21). At the conclusion of the program with 2796 patients, cumulative AE sensitivity is 1.1/1000. There are many potential AE types that would occur at a rate of 1/100,000 and thus the need for postmarket surveillance to clarify the safety profile of the drug.

Table A.1 in the Appendix presents a table of adverse events observed in placebo-controlled trials for marketed drugs together with the number of patients enrolled on each treatment arm. The list reveals that the adverse events observed are the most common and not necessarily most serious. The postmarket phase will reveal the rare and potentially serious adverse events. We will revisit this table again in various chapters.

Lin, Chern, and Chu (2003) acknowledge this limitation but are concerned that failure to find cases of liver toxicity in a confirmatory trial might lead to a conclusion that the experimental drug is not associated with liver toxicity. They provide useful guidelines for surrogates, such as laboratory values, to liver disease that might be uncovered in a clinical trial. DMC members can, presumably, discuss surrogates for other diseases when appropriate.

Postmarket experience will be needed to uncover SAEs that occur with low incidence. The clinical programs generally enroll patients with much narrower characteristics than for those who will receive the drug after approval. Eligibility requirements specify strict age groups, and prohibit enrollment of patients with certain medical histories, comorbidities, and concurrent medications. As larger numbers and newer types of patients are exposed to the drug postapproval newer SAEs are likely to emerge. In the postapproval era, papers appear in the literature presenting safety profiles of drugs using over many controlled clinical trials. Examples would include Schoenfeld (1999) for gastrointestinal safety of the nonsteroidal anti-inflammatory drug meloxicam, Strampel, Emkey, and Civitelli (2007) for the safety profile of bisphosphonates in the treatment of osteoporosis, and Wernicke, Lledo, Raskin et al. (2007) for the cardiovascular safety profile of duloxetine used to treat major depressive disorder. A summary of limitations of a clinical program to uncover important safety issues is presented in Table 1.4.

TABLE 1.4

Limitations of Safety Assessment by a DMC in a Single Clinical Trial

1. DMC is likely to find only AEs that occur immediately and with highest frequency.
2. DMC not likely to find rare or delayed effects.
3. DMC may not develop an understanding of chronic effects.
4. Due to stringent eligibility requirements, clinical trial patients are not representative of those who will be treated with the drug after approval. Different patient types on varying concomitant medications may have a different but more common safety experience than the clinical trial patients.
5. DMC may miss subtle signals that involve extensive analysis and additional data on surrogates of AEs.

1.6.3 Postmarket Safety Actions

After FDA approves a drug, there are several actions the agency may take when safety concerns arise. These actions include ordering the drug withdrawn from the market, attaching a *black box warning* to the drug's package insert (i.e., label change to highlight the description of the SAE in the package insert), and ordering discontinuation of a dosage form. Carpenter, Zucker, and Avorn (2008) report that during the period 1993–2004, FDA made 11 safety-based withdrawals and 14 black box warnings (21 drugs had either a withdrawal or black box warning or both) and 36 had dosage form discontinuation. Lasser, Allen, Woolhandler et al. (2002) indicate that there were 548 new chemical entities approved by FDA during the period 1975–1999 and of these, 56 drugs (10.2%) acquired a black box warning or were withdrawn. On the basis of the FDA's adverse experience reporting system during the period 1969–2002, a total of 75 drugs or drug products were removed and 11 received restricted prescription requirements (Wysowski and Swartz 2005). Table 1.5 presents a partial list of drugs withdrawn from the market for safety reasons during the period 1975–2007.

Of the 740 new molecular entities approved by FDA in 1980–2009, only 26 were withdrawn for safety reasons (3.5%). An additional 92 products were withdrawn for other reasons. The frequency of safety withdrawals decreased from 50% of withdrawals in the 1980s, 40% in the 1990s to 10% in the 2000s (Quereshi, Seoane-Vazquez, Rodriquez-Monguio et al. 2011).

Lasser, Allen, Woolhandler et al. (2002) list 28 drugs for which black box warnings were issued during the period 1975–2000. The timing of the warnings ranged from 1- to 23-year postapproval. The frequency of black box warnings appears to have accelerated since 2000 with adverse events of new awareness and interest and new sources of safety evidence. For example, since 2000, 50 drugs received black box warnings for suicide risk (Mundy 2008). Rosiglitazone, indicated for diabetes, received a black box warning for cardiovascular risk with much of the evidence coming from a meta-analysis published by an academic cardiologist (Harris 2007; Nissen and Wolski 2007).

There is a considerable controversy about the timing and appropriateness of specific postapproval drug actions (Friedman, Woodcock, Lumpkin et al. 1999; Lurie and Sasich 1999; Lasser, Allen, Woolhandler et al. 2002; Carpenter, Zucker, and Avorn 2008). Much of this controversy stems from a misunderstanding of the extent that a clinical program can reveal safety concerns and the differences of opinion in the ability and methodology to assess early safety signals from clinical trials. The following chapters will explain how DMCs can help in identification of safety signals.

1.6.4 Role of DMCs in Exploratory and Confirmatory Trials

This book will concentrate on DMCs in confirmatory trials where they are used most frequently. There is no doubt that there is a need for safety

TABLE 1.5

Partial List of Drugs Withdrawn from the Market for Safety Reasons, 1977–2007

Drug	Indication/Class	Risks	Approved	Withdrawn
Aprotinin	Reduce blood loss during cardiovascular surgery	Complications of surgery; death	1998	2007
Pergolide	Parkinson's disease	Heart valve damage	1988	2007
Tegaserod maleate	Irritable bowel syndrome	Myocardial infarct; stroke	2002	2008
Valdecoxib	Pain, anti-inflammatory	Heart attack, stroke	2001	2005
Rofecoxib	Pain	Thrombotic events	1999	2004
Cerivastatin	Lipid lowering	Muscle damage	1997	2001
Rapacuronium bromide	Injectable anesthetic	Bronchospasm	1999	2001
Alosetron	Irritable bowel syndrome in women	Intestinal damage	2000	2000
Cisapride	Night heartburn	Fatal heart rhythm	1993	2000
Troglitazone	Type 2 diabetes	Severe liver toxicity	1997	2000
Astemizole	Antihistamine	Fatal heart rhythm	1988	1999
Grepafloxacin	Antibiotic	Fatal heart rhythm	1997	1999
Mibefradil	High blood pressure and chronic stable angina	Dangerous interactions with other drugs	1997	1998
Bromfenac	Pain	Severe liver damage	1997	1998
Terfenadine	Antihistamine	Fatal heart rhythm	1985	1998
Fenfluramine	Obesity	Heart valve abnormalities	1973	1997
Dexfenfluramine	Obesity	Heart valve abnormalities	1996	1997
Flosequinan	Cardiovascular disease	Increased mortality	1992	1993
Temafloxacin	Antibiotic	Hemolytic anemia, renal failure, and so on	1992	1992
Encainide	Antiarrhythmic	Increased mortality	1986	1991
Nomifensine	Antidepressant	Hemolytic anemia	1984	1986
Suprofen	Analgesic, NSAID[a]	Pain	1984	1986
Zomepirac	Analgesic, NSAID[a]	Anaphylaxis	1980	1983
Benoxaprofen	Analgesic, NSAID[a]	Jaundice	1982	1982
Ticrynafen	Antihypertensive	Hepatic toxicity	1979	1980
Azarbine	Psoriasis	Thromboembolism	1975	1977

Source: U.S. Food and Drug Administration. 2002. Safety-based drug withdrawals (1997–2001), http://www.fda.gov/Safety/Recalls/ArchiveRecalls/default.htm; Lasser, K. E. et al. 2002. *Journal of American Medical Association,* **287**, 2215–2220; FOI Services. 2008. Document search, www.foiservices.com.

[a] Nonsteroidal anti-inflammatory drug.

monitoring in exploratory trials especially since these represent the first use of new drugs in humans. However, it is not clear that this must be accomplished through a completely independent DMC and many feel that engaging a completely independent committee would at this stage slow down the development process. In a paper commissioned by the Society for Clinical Trials, Dixon, Freedman, Herson et al. (2006) give useful guidance on this issue as do Hibberd and Weiner (2004).

The phase I trial uses objective safety data and the protocol team in-house together with participating investigators who can generally handle the safety monitoring with little question of credibility. Phase II does not usually require a completely independent DMC but it often makes sense to include one or two outside members (physician or physician plus biostatistician) to the protocol team with the understanding that one of the outside people will take the role of Chair of the DMC when the drug enters confirmatory trials. This allows for some outside expertise in the first efficacy trials and provides drug familiarity for the confirmatory DMC. Of course, if the trial is first for a novel drug such as a drug-eluting stent or one utilizing gene therapy or nanotechnology, it may be advisable to add to the DMC additional outside reviewers with the particular expertise.

1.6.5 Blurring of Phases I, II, and III

Regulators have become concerned about the recent use of Phase Ib expansion protocols in oncology. One trial that caught their eye is the KEYNOTE-001 trial for the PD-1 inhibitor pembrolizumab (Patnaik, Kang, Rasco et al. 2015) which was initiated in 2011 to determine a dose for phase II trials in advanced solid tumors. As favorable responses were observed, the sample size increased and different tumor types were added until there were over 1200 patients on this Phase 1b protocol. Among these, there were 173 patients with advanced melanoma and this was considered sufficient for accelerated approval. However, as the number of patients increased the sponsor did not add a DMC. Had development progressed in the traditional phase I, II, and III sequence, there would certainly have been a DMC for the confirmatory trial.

1.6.6 Investigator-Sponsored Trials

In the United States, investigator-sponsored trials are those conducted by an academic physician (investigator) using drugs provided by a pharmaceutical company. The investigator, rather than the sponsor, is responsible for all interaction with FDA. Thus, sponsors have little control over investigator-sponsored trials but there is clearly a need for safety review. When the investigator-sponsored trial is conducted within a single institution and that institution has a standing internal DMC to monitor trials that do not otherwise have a DMC, this body would usually be sufficient. If no such panel exists or the trial is multicenter, investigators might want to consider some of the ideas for exploratory trials above.

1.6.7 Open Label Trials

A clinical trial needn't be masked to require a DMC. Trials for mechanical heart valves, for example, are uncontrolled yet have serious safety problems such as major bleeding events, thromboembolic events, and mortality (Grunkenmeier, Jin, and Starr 2006). It is important that there be independent review of accumulating data. In Chapter 3, we will describe how these meetings are conducted.

For chronic conditions such as epilepsy, Parkinson's disease, and hypertension, it is common for patients who exit phase II or III trials to be put on open label extension studies. These trials are uncontrolled and have the purpose of obtaining more precision in estimation of incidence of adverse events and, perhaps, to uncover new adverse events encountered in long-term exposure. DMCs may be asked to review data from ongoing open label extension studies while they are reviewing data from controlled trials. At the very least, the DMC should review the extension study results at the end of the final confirmatory trial. Day and Williams (2007) provide insight in the role of the open label extension study in drug development.

1.6.8 Emerging Trial Designs of Interest

As the pace of drug development accelerates, much attention has been drawn to pragmatic trials, biosimilar trials, SMART/dynamic treatment strategy trials, umbrella trials, and basket trials. We will explain the role of DMCs in these trials in Chapter 8, after we get further grounding in DMC operations. For now, it is safe to say that these types of trials, although they present certain challenges, all require independent review of accumulating data.

1.7 Pharmaceutical Industry Demographics

1.7.1 Size of Companies

For the purposes of this book, the global pharmaceutical/biotechnology industry will be divided into three gross size groups. The term "Big Pharma" will apply to multinational companies that have many products in development and many products on the market either as recently approved or generic. "Middle Pharma" will refer to companies with just a few products on the market and several in development. Those companies working in the development of their first product will be called "Infant Pharma."

1.7.2 Public versus Private Companies

All of the Big Pharma companies and most of the Middle Pharma companies are publicly owned. Many of the Infant Pharma firms are publicly owned and those that are financed by venture capital firms seeking to raise additional rounds of financing while pursuing an exit strategy which would consist of taking the company public or selling it to a larger company. Today's reality is that, regardless of size, these companies are vulnerable to information that must be reported to investors on company activities and especially R&D (research and development) activities. Actions taken by DMCs can affect the financial status of these companies although differently depending on size. We will return to this important topic at various times in this book. For purposes of contrast, we will be referring to Big versus Infant Pharma in much of what follows. As would be expected, Middle Pharma shares some characteristics of both its big and little brothers. Middle Pharma is very dependent on Big Pharma as a marketing partner for their products and for investment in R&D programs. Middle firms are very dependent on public markets for financing their new products. If a Middle Pharma firm has not had a product approved since it emerged from infancy and has had a string of disappointments since emerging, it would be highly vulnerable to DMC negative decisions. The differences in the three levels of companies are further described in Table 1.6.

TABLE 1.6

Characteristics of Pharmaceutical/Biotechnology Companies by Size

Characteristic	Big Pharma	Middle Pharma	Infant Pharma
Products on the market	Many products on the market	Some products on the market	None
Financial organization	Public	Public	Public or venture capital financed
Corporate goal	Expand product line	Expand product line; create corporate partnerships with Big Pharma	Show progress to increase financing, license the product to the larger company
Clinical program financing	Complete	Almost complete	Trial-by-trial basis, further funding for pivotal trial might depend on the results of interim analysis
Vulnerability to negative trial information	Small, unless the drug is the successor to the blockbuster	Modest, especially vulnerable if it has been some time since the last product was approved	Considerable
DMC procedures	In place	In place	Not well developed, often created as the trial develops

1.8 In Conclusion

We have now seen the rationale and the setting for DMCs in the pharmaceutical industry. In the next chapter, we will learn more about the members of the safety monitoring team and their roles.

DMCounselor

Q1.1 I agreed to serve on a DMC for an Infant Pharma company which has gone public. The drug is a novel approach to pancreatic cancer. The trial is actually phase II but their regulatory consultant feels that if the results are positive, the regulatory agency will consider it phase III. The sponsor has now told us that we will meet only once at the end of the trial because their board of directors is concerned that if we recommend early trial termination due to a safety concern, they would have to include this information in a press release and this would have a bad effect on their stock price. I would like to walk away from this DMC but this is an important drug and I would like to be associated with its development. What should I do?

A I had doubts about this sponsor when I heard that they have a consultant who told them that a phase II trial would count as a phase III trial in this case. It is doubtful that sufficient safety data would arise in a single phase II trial. In any case, this sponsor's restrictions do not allow the DMC to fill the stewardship role. It is the DMC's responsibility to decide how often they will meet, not the sponsor's. The DMC must review accumulated data during the trial so that patients are not put at risk for a trial's duration if serious concerns arise during the trial. If this sponsor is afraid of an interim recommendation, why would they want a DMC to make an assessment at the end of the trial? You should try to convince the sponsor not to begin the phase II/III until they have more confidence in the safety of this product. At that point, there should be much less financial risk in having a DMC schedule periodic meetings during the trial.

Q1.2 I was asked to serve on a DMC for a phase II trial. I said that I would do so provided I would automatically be placed on the DMC for the phase III trial. The sponsor refused. Why would they do this?

A The sponsor was right in this instance. While it is a good idea to have some continuity between phase II and phase III, it is also good to have some new people on the phase III trials. In choosing which, if any, phase II DMC members would carry over to the phase III DMC sponsors would usually wait until the phase II trial was concluded at which time they would have learned from that trial what type of expertise was needed for the phase III DMC.

Q1.3 I was asked to serve as a biostatistician member of a DMC. I accepted and found out that the trial was phase I. Is a biostatistician member really needed for a phase I trial?

A Outside members are not usually employed on phase I trials but the sponsor appears to think that it is necessary in this case. Do not think that you are not needed just because you will not be looking at confidence intervals and explaining survival curves to the physician members? Your knowledge of protocols, objectivity, logical thinking, and so on, would be very important to the committee.

Q1.4 I was asked to be a physician member of a DMC for a neurology drug by a Middle Pharma company. I accepted but later found out that the trial was completed 5 months ago without a DMC. The sponsor is now in negotiations to license the drug to a Big Pharma company and the latter insists that there be an independent review of safety before talks can continue. Is this an appropriate use of my time?

A The committee the sponsor is forming is not a data *monitoring* committee but an ad hoc committee to come in once and make statements about safety presumably by also taking efficacy into account. This committee will obviously be unmasked and will not have had the benefit of considering and scrutinizing safety issues as they arise. If you feel you want to serve, this is OK but make sure that the sponsor does not represent your committee as a DMC. The sponsor must also understand that your committee is not coming together for 2 hours to be a "rubber stamp" on safety. If your committee needs more time and information it must be granted. Also, your committee should not be brought to the table either as individuals or collectively to be part of business negotiations with the company purchasing the license.

Q1.5 I am a physician member of an Infant Pharma co. trial of a new agent for interstitial bladder cancer. This is my first participation in a pharmaceutical industry DMC. I have about 10 years of experience working on DMCs sponsored by NIH. The DMC has been meeting several times over the past 18 months. In that time, there has been an ongoing Securities Exchange Commission investigation of the sponsor, the chief executive officer (CEO) has resigned and left the country, we are now on our third vice president (VP)–chief medical officer, and each time the medical officer resigns, the two or three clinical operations staff members leave as well. Is this typical of Infant Pharma? How can I tell if I am wasting my time on this?

A These things do occur in Infant Pharma but I am not aware of occurrences to this extent. I understand your concern and the culture shock you must be feeling. However, I think you must separate the officers of the company from the actual trial operations. In spite of the turnover, are you getting data of reasonable quality to examine? Do you have any evidence of fraudulent data? I would expect the clinical operations to be separate from the corporate-level problems. This would especially be the case if a CRO (contract research organization) were running the trial. I would encourage you to discuss your concern with the other DMC members and your DMC Chair should indicate that the DMC has a concern with the turnover among clinical operations staff. No, I do not think you are wasting your time.

2

Organization of a Safety Monitoring Program for a Confirmatory Trial

PREVIEW   The independence of a data monitoring committee (DMC) from the sponsor must be preserved and even the appearance of conflict of interest must be avoided. The Data Analysis Center (DAC) is the organization that will prepare the data for DMC review. The DAC is preferably, but not always, independent of the sponsor. The sponsor's standard operating procedures (SOPs) should cover the creation and operations of the DMC. The typical DMC has three members—two physicians and a biostatistician. All three are voting members. The biostatistician from the DAC is a nonvoting member. Other committees involved in confirmatory trial review are described.

KEY WORDS: *independence, conflict of interest, Data Analysis Center (DAC), contract research organization (CRO), institutional review board (IRB), endpoint adjudication committee, steering committee*

2.1 Members of the Safety Monitoring Team

2.1.1 The Sponsor

As was indicated earlier, the *sponsor* is the organization that pays for the trial and whose objective is to get the experimental drug approved by regulatory agencies. The sponsor will have the task of appointing a DMC before the start of the clinical trial and ensuring its independence. An important person within the sponsor organization is the *sponsor representative* to the DMC. This person is typically the senior clinical research professional in charge of the trial. This person will coordinate sponsor activities and those of the other elements of the safety monitoring operation. The person will generally be in charge of a protocol team of people who will work with the DMC. These team members will generally represent clinical operations, biostatistics, data management, and safety surveillance. The sponsor representative might possess an MD, PhD, or PharmD. However, regardless of degree, this individual will have the clinical research experience necessary to be leading the trial. In Infant Pharma, the sponsor representative might be the vice president, clinical research/medical director of the company or it might be a person with extensive clinical operations experience because the person acting as medical director is a contract consultant to the sponsor. In Big Pharma and Middle Pharma, the sponsor representative will mention several people above them in the organization that have responsibility for the therapeutic area and the trial at hand. It will be important for the DMC members and especially the Chair to understand who the DMC reports to under different circumstances.

There are many characteristics for a sponsor representative that would be considered desirable. The most important is that the sponsor recognizes the DMC as being responsible for the stewardship of the trial and being independent of the sponsor. Table 2.1 presents a list of desirable characteristics for a sponsor representative. The rationale for many items on this list will become more obvious in later chapters of this book.

2.1.2 Data Monitoring Committee

The DMC is the subject of this book. Much more will be said about its composition and functions later. For now, it is sufficient to reinforce the DMC is an *independent* committee of individuals, with credentials in medicine, biostatistics, and so on, who are not employees of the sponsor or investigators/biostatisticians on the trial having the responsibility of stewardship for the trial. In this capacity, the committee will protect patient safety by periodic review of safety data and responding to trends in serious adverse events whenever they may occur. DMCs also have efficacy and risk–benefit responsibilities and these will be covered in subsequent chapters.

TABLE 2.1

Desirable Characteristics in a Sponsor Representative to the DMC

---

1. Respect the DMC as being responsible for the stewardship of the trial and remember that the DMC members are at least partially unmasked to treatment and sponsor staff is completely masked.
2. Respect the independence of the DMC.
3. Interact and respect the views of the entire committee not just the Chair or the person of a certain discipline.
4. Respect the views of other sponsor staff especially with their interactions with DMC members of the same discipline.
5. Be open minded about DMC requests for ad hoc computer programming, consultants, and so on, but not intimidated about asking for justification.
6. Knowledgeable about clinical trial operations in general and those of the CRO and DAC that may be involved in this trial.
7. Knowledge of sponsor SOPs for DMCs, the DMC Charter, and FDA/ICH guidelines for DMCs and safety reporting.
8. Knowledgeable about the clinical issues in the disease being treated, experimental drug, its safety profile, and clinical trial history.
9. Knowledge of statistics as applied to clinical trials.

2.1.3 Data Analysis Center

The *Data Analysis Center (DAC)* is the organization that will prepare tables and reports to the DMC under formats requested by the DMC. The DAC could be the statistical unit of the sponsor or a CRO. A biostatistician from the DAC will be called the *independent statistician* and will be a nonvoting ex officio member of the DMC. The DAC will have the treatment assignment codes and, thus, members can unmask themselves at any time. It is thus preferable that the DAC will not be the same organization working on the ultimate regulatory submission. However, sponsors and CROs working on the regulatory submissions have found satisfactory ways of building a "firewall" between those providing DAC services and those working on the regulatory submissions. Much has been written about the need for independence or ways of constructing this firewall (see, e.g., Ellenberg and George 2004; Siegel, O'Neil, Temple et al. 2004; Snapinn, Cook, Shapiro et al. 2004). Nevertheless, the degree of independence that actually exists in any situation remains a controversial topic. More will be said about the DAC and its place in data flow later.

In addition to statistical analysis, DACs sometimes perform administrative functions such as making travel arrangements and paying DMC members. However, DACs should be chosen on their ability to support safety surveillance in an ongoing clinical trial, not primarily on the basis of computer programming or administrative abilities. A list of desirable characteristics for a DAC will be found in Table 2.2.

In some clinical trials, especially those run in Europe, the biostatistician member of the DMC is given safety dataset prior to the DMC meeting and this individual prepares the data for review and performs all other functions that the DAC biostatistician would normally perform. There is

TABLE 2.2

Desirable Characteristics for a Data Analysis Center (DAC)

1. Experience in serving as a DAC
2. SOPs for DAC operations
3. SOPs for software validation
4. Knowledge of FDA and ICH guidelines for safety reporting and data monitoring committees
5. Knowledge of MedDRA (Medical Dictionary for Regulatory Affairs, see Chapter 4) coding of AEs
6. Library of validated software for report generation and statistical analysis
7. Flexible staff for timely response to ad hoc requests
8. If needed by sponsor can the DAC support administrative services such as travel and meeting arrangements, and host conference calls?
9. Off-site computer backup
10. Statistical staff with knowledge of
    a. Clinical trial statistical methods
    b. Interim analysis methodology including conditional power, predictive power (these terms will be defined in Chapter 5)

no problem with this approach but, in what follows, we will assume that the DMC is working with a separate DAC biostatistician. In trials where the DAC biostatistician has responsibility for preparing tables and doing statistical analysis, it is important to decide, at the outset, if the DMC biostatistician member can also receive data to do additional ad hoc analyses. The cost control issues and procedures of such a practice must also be discussed before the trial begins.

2.1.4 Institutional Review Board

An *Institutional Review Board* (IRB) exists at every institution performing medical or behavioral research in human subjects in the United States. IRBs are regulated by FDA and the Office for Human Research Protections in the Department of Health and Human Services (Code of Federal Regulations 2016). In other parts of the world, similar committees are often referred to as ethics committees. The IRBs are responsible for reviewing proposed and ongoing research at their institutions to decide if the research is ethical, informed consent is sufficient, and appropriate safeguards, such as the existence of a DMC, are in place. IRBs review protocols and their amendments, investigator brochures, serious adverse event reports, and so on. There is some overlap with DMCs but the DMC is responsible for the stewardship of the trial over all institutions while the IRBs have responsibility within their institution. The DMC reviews all trial safety data on a regular basis, can be unmasked but receives at least partially masked data, and can recommend termination of the trial. The IRB reviews only trial-wide serious adverse events that are serious, drug related, and unexpected. The IRB also reviews an annual report of SAEs judged to be related to drug and can recommend termination of the trial at their institution.

We will see that DMCs review more information than IRBs but they should certainly review no less. A summary of IRB and DMC roles in safety surveillance is presented in Table 2.3.

2.1.5 Other Committees That Might Be Involved

Some confirmatory clinical trials will have *endpoint adjudication committees* and *steering committees*. The endpoint adjudication committee will review images, EKGs, hematology, and so on, to determine if a patient's clinical endpoints have been attained. They typically have at least three members and they review their data masked to treatment assignment. The steering committee's role will vary from sponsor to sponsor and trial to trial. They are essentially an advisory committee on the conduct of the trial. While the DMC and the endpoint adjudication committees must remain as independent of the sponsor as possible, the steering committee can and should be advocates for the sponsor's product. It is important to minimize misunderstandings on overlapping responsibilities and the hierarchy of decision making. It will be

TABLE 2.3

Safety Monitoring by Institutional Review Boards versus Data Monitoring Committees

Characteristics	IRB	DMC
Origin	Required by law in most countries	Recommended by regulatory agencies for phase III clinical trials
Purpose	Big picture—ethics and safety, at institutional level	Detailed safety review trialwide
Review expedited adverse events (serious, possibly related, and unexpected)	Yes	Yes
Other adverse events	Annual update of related	Frequent update of all adverse events
Treatment group information	No	Yes
Review: protocol	Yes	Yes
Investigator brochure	Yes	Yes
Informed consent	Review and approve	Review but not approve

very important that each committee understands its objectives and relationship with other committees especially if a hierarchy exists or is implied. In Chapter 3, we will learn the details of a DMC Charter. Similarly, the endpoint adjudication committee and the steering committee will have charters and these charters will ideally explain the responsibilities and boundaries. It would be considered good practice for the Chair of each committee to have a copy of the charters of the other committees so that he/she can refer to them should a jurisdictional question arise.

2.1.6 Scope of DMC Authority

DMC opinions on safety are advisory to the sponsor. It should not be assumed that if a sponsor and DMC are in agreement that there are no serious safety issues that the drug is now automatically classified as safe. The regulatory agencies will have the final say in this matter.

2.2 How Is a DMC Created?

The sponsor has the responsibility for creating the DMC. This is generally done as soon as most investigators are selected and it is clear that certain physicians who could serve as investigators will not be serving as such. This latter group would serve as a pool for selection of physician DMC members. Ideally the DMC should be in place before the first patient is randomized to the trial. Unfortunately, this is not always the case (see *DMCounselor* Q2.2 below). Typically, the sponsor's study team would meet to go down a list of candidates, prioritize them, and then begin contacting candidates from the top of the list.

All activities for the creation, organization, and management of DMCs should be covered in the sponsor's standard operating procedures (SOPs). These SOPs would typically be found as part of SOPs for the sponsor's over- all risk management plan (Haas 2004; Bush, Dai, Dieck et al. 2005). More will be said of SOPs for DMCs later but it is important to note here that, like many drug development activities, sponsor staff should not be forming a DMC by intuition but rather by following documented procedures. The need for DMC SOPs applies to all sponsors regardless of size. However, experience shows that Big Pharma and Middle Pharma have SOPs in place and most of their clinical staff members are well versed in, or at least familiar with, these procedures. Infant Pharma companies are often creating procedures as they go along partly because of time constraints and partly because of the need to create a balance between differing procedures that staff bring with them from their former companies. This can sometimes be frustrating for DMC members but it should be looked at as an opportunity to help the start-up create the best procedures.

The principal organizational document for the DMC is the DMC Charter. The charter is an outgrowth of the SOPs and indicates the responsibilities of all parties within and outside the DMC. More will be said about the DMC Charter in the next chapter.

2.3 Membership

Let's now consider some of the characteristics appropriate and not appropri- ate for DMC members.

2.3.1 Physicians

The physician members will be of two types—those with expertise in the indication under investigation and those with expertise in expected adverse events. In a trial for rheumatoid arthritis, we would certainly want to include rheumatologists who specialize in rheumatoid arthritis. However, if it is known that cardiovascular events (moderate hypertension, transient arrhythmia) are likely a cardiologist might be included. For a drug used to treat diabetic shock, a diabetes specialist would be needed but also, perhaps, an emergency medicine expert. In multiregional trials, it is advisable to include physicians who practice in the various cultures. These members can fill the usual physician role as well as advise on cultural issues that might affect the nature of adverse event reports. More will be said about DMC issues in multiregional trials in Chapter 4.

2.3.2 Biostatisticians

A biostatistician will serve on the DMC. This person should be experienced in the indication for the trial and familiar with statistical methods for safety analysis as well as efficacy analysis. If innovative methods of design and analysis are to be employed (e.g., adaptive designs, Bayesian methods), the biostatistical member should be well versed in these techniques and be able to explain them to the physician members.

2.3.3 How Many Members Are Needed?

While three members—two physicians and a biostatistician—appears to be the norm the precise number needed depends on the complexity of the trial and the various kinds of expertise needed. Suffice it to say that the number of members should be the minimal needed to cover the waterfront of expertise. DMCs with more than one biostatistician are rare. As mentioned above, the DAC will contribute their own biostatistician to the committee as a nonvoting member. As we will see later, scheduling DMC meetings is not easy even when they are done as telephone conference calls. The more people the more difficult it is to schedule meetings. If there was a five-person committee on an oncology trial with one of the people being a neurologist as an AE expert (i.e., neurological AEs expected), and three members present constituting a quorum, it is possible that the trial could run to completion with the neurologist never attending a meeting and this input would be marginalized. Of course, meetings should be scheduled so that no member misses the meeting. The quorum rule should only be invoked because a member must not attend due to a last-minute emergency. Even then, the DMC Chair can get input from the absent parties over the next few days after the meeting.

2.3.4 Ad Hoc Consultants

One way to keep a DMC at a reasonable size is to add ad hoc consultants when issues arise requiring expertise not present on the committee. For example, it might make more sense to bring an allergist in to consult on hypersensitivity events than to have this person as a sitting member of the committee. While ethicists and patient advocates are often present as DMC members on trials sponsored by the NIH (Friedman and DeMets 1981), they would usually appear as consultants in pharmaceutical trials except for those trials where serious ethical issues occur regularly. An example of the latter in the field of psychiatric drugs would be in mood disorders (Charney, Nemeroff, Lewis et al. 2002). Recent examples in medical devices would include vagus nerve stimulators for depression (Rush, Marangell, Sackheim et al. 2005; Schuchman 2007) and extracorporeal liver assist devices (Ellis, Hughes, Wendon et al. 1996). Sponsors generally rely on IRBs for input on the "big picture" ethical issues.

2.3.5 Ubiquitous DMC Members

It is best not to appoint people to a DMC who are currently serving on multiple DMCs, say five or more. Often-used members may confuse issues and protocols between the various trials and it is good to have many different people serving on DMCs instead of creating a power elite. Service on a DMC is confidential so that sponsors must rely on the judgment of potential DMC members in this regard.

It is reasonable for those who have not served on DMCs before to be unsure about serving when first asked. Table 2.4 presents a list of useful questions that potential DMC members might ask a sponsor before agreeing to serve on a DMC. Those using this table should beware of vague answers or promises to find answers that are not fulfilled in a timely manner. As a DMC member, you will be on a committee responsible for the stewardship of the trial, similar to being a board of directors of the trial. In speaking to the sponsor representative, it is important to ascertain if the sponsor sees the DMC with this responsibility or does this person see it as merely a necessary

TABLE 2.4

Questions to Ask a Sponsor before Agreeing to Serve on a Data Monitoring Committee

---

1. Look over the clinical trial protocol and draft the DMC Charter.
2. Who will the other members be, either by name or specialization?
3. Will contract include indemnification?
4. When does the trial begin?
5. How many meetings are proposed per year, how many are face-to-face?
6. What type of adverse events are expected, what severity?
7. Will the DMC be responsible for efficacy or just safety?
8. Will the DMC be asked to comment on manuscripts reporting trial results before submission to journals?
9. If asked to Chair the DMC
   a. Is there a budget for ad hoc requests to the DAC?
   b. Who in sponsor management do I report to?
   c. Will the DMC have the freedom to design tables for review of safety or must the committee use tables already designed by the sponsor?
   d. If Internet interactive software is to be used by DMC members how will training be handled? What are the resources for support/troubleshooting?
   e. Who are the other members of the DMC and by what process were they selected?
   f. In what countries will the trial be conducted?
   g. Will there be a central clinical laboratory for all centers?
   h. On what criteria was the DAC selected? What are their capabilities?

---

appendage like certain clauses in an informed consent form. Any evidence of the latter should be treated with caution.

Similarly, a potential DMC member may be unsure if he/she is the right person to be serving on a DMC. Table 2.5 presents questions that the potential DMC might ponder to help decide if DMC service is right for them at least at this time. This table might also serve as a checklist for sponsors interviewing potential DMC members.

2.3.6 Disclosure of DMC Membership

The protocol for the trial should indicate the existence of a DMC but there does not appear to be any advantage to disclosing the names of the members of a DMC to investigators or the public at large until the trial is completed. If the identity of the members is known during the trial, investigators, competitors, or others might attempt to extract information about trial progress from them in informal settings.

2.3.7 Multiple Sponsorship

In diseases such as cancer, human immunodeficiency virus (HIV), malaria, and so on, it is not unusual for the pharmaceutical industry sponsor to have cosponsors such as National Cancer Institute or other NIH component, World Health Organization, Gates Foundation, Cooperative Oncology Groups, and so on. These organizations may have existing committees that have functions similar to pharmaceutical industry DMCs and feel that these committees are sufficient to meet DMC requirements. Sponsors should make sure that all of their SOPs and regulatory requirements will be achieved by the existing committee (see *DMCounselor Q2.3* below).

TABLE 2.5

Questions for an Individual to Ponder before Agreeing to Serve on a Data Monitoring Committee

---

1. Is your primary interest in protecting patient safety (+) or earning a consulting fee (−)?
2. Do you have the time to devote to DMC service including flexibility for ad hoc emergency meetings (+)?
3. Do you like working on committees (+)?
4. Do you appreciate the interdisciplinary and multicultural nature of clinical trials (+) or do you tend to feel that people would agree with you if they only had the same training and background that you have (−)?
5. Do you feel that even though the sponsor is paying you a fee that you can remain independent of the sponsor (+)?
6. If asked to Chair a DMC
   a. Are you a consensus builder (+) or do you feel that as Chair you have the final say (−)?
   b. Do you have the time to get the committee together for ad hoc meetings, review ad hoc meeting material, and to continually interact with sponsor staff on DMC matters (+)?

Note: +indicates favorable trait, −indicates negative trait.

2.3.8 From Where Are DMC Members Recruited?

Typically, DMC members come from the ranks of academia, government, nonprofit organizations, and semi or fully-retired professionals. Members may serve on DMCs for several sponsors simultaneously as long as no conflict of interest is seen.

Some sponsors are selecting patient advocates as full DMC members. These are patients who have been treated with the same class of drug and/ or have had the same disease as the patients in the trial but are not patients on the current trial. The patient advocate can present the patient's point of view on safety issues. The patient advocate might have a different perspective on adverse events that might be viewed as "acceptable" to physician and biostatistical DMC members.

2.4 Term

The usual term for DMC members is one trial or two trials if the two are being run simultaneously to satisfy regulatory requirements of submitting "at least one well-controlled trial" for marketing approval. While there is a definite advantage to retain one clinical person through several trials—phase II, III, and IIIB—many sponsors avoid creating a "Supreme Court" where the same DMC serves throughout the lifetime of the product because of the advantages of getting different points of view and the danger that some members may make decisions on drug safety in early trials and not pay proper attention to new information in confirmatory trials. However, there is nothing wrong in an ethical or regulatory sense with the same people serving throughout.

2.5 Conflicts of Interest and DMC Independence from Sponsor

Justice Potter Stewart once said "I can't define pornography but I know it when I see it" (U.S. Supreme Court 1964). Similarly, conflict of interest for DMC members cannot be precisely defined but, as was said in Chapter 1, persuasiveness of results requires that even the appearance of conflict of interest must be avoided. Sponsor SOPs should provide conflict of interest guidelines. These guidelines should require financial disclosure of equity interest in the sponsor or those with competing products, consulting, and/ or investigator arrangements with the sponsor or competitors, proprietary interest in the drug under investigation or competing products. For some products, such as orphan drugs, the diseases are so rare there may be only one or two physicians with appropriate expertise to serve on a DMC. In these cases, joint service must be allowed under the condition that the sponsor will not use the opportunity to find out information about a competitor's clinical program and that the DMC member will not divulge information about the competitor.

There will always be debate about whether or not the DMC is truly independent of the sponsor and how independence can be achieved (Fleming, Hennekens, Pfeffer et al. 2014) but following some reasonable steps should ensure that its members are at least more independent of the outcome of the trial than the sponsor.

Sponsor SOPs should require some level of financial disclosure prior to finalizing appointment to a DMC. DMC members should not have sizable consulting contracts with the sponsor at the time of DMC service. Sponsor SOPs should include a cutoff in dollars as to what is sizable. This cutoff would be of advantage to Infant Pharma because it will minimize the chance of thier getting into a bidding war with Big Pharma for available talent.

Asking if a DMC can be independent of sponsor is like asking if elected officials can be independent of their major campaign donors or if media companies can be independent of their advertisers. These entanglements are due to financial arrangements. In Chapter 8, we will explore the possibility of DMCs being compensated not by the sponsors whose clinical trials they are monitoring but by a third party, perhaps FDA. In the meantime, so much of the perception of independence depends on the attitude of the DMC Chair. A Chair who runs meetings as if the DMC is independent is much better than one who looks to the sponsor to decide agendas, run meetings, and so on. The latter type of Chair often arises when he/she is selected by the sponsor prior to the first meeting of the DMC. Having the DMC members elect a member from those present at the orientation meeting might appear as a good strategy but in Chapter 3 we will see why this is not practical.

2.6 Compensation

The level of compensation that DMC members receive for their service is closely related to conflict of interest. There is the perception that if DMC members were paid too well they would be less independent of the sponsor. Sponsors should have guidelines for reasonable compensation and this is a matter that can be discussed among sponsors. In multiregional trials, the DMC will usually consist of members from different countries and the definition of reasonable compensation will differ among countries. As long as compensation levels are not extravagant, Infant Pharma can afford to retain the same professionals for DMC service as Big Pharma. Of course, compensation should not be so low that members cannot justify taking the time to do the necessary work away from their "day jobs." DMC members should think of this activity as a service to drug development and not as a lucrative consulting sideline.

2.7 Liability and Indemnification

Physician members of DMCs are serving as consultants to the sponsor and, thus, are not covered by malpractice insurance that may be in force at the institutions where they practice. The same would apply to biostatisticians. All DMC members should be responsible for intentional negligence but indemnification has emerged as a standard way to protect DMC members against liabilities that arise in the trial for which they are not responsible. Confusion arises when a sponsor's legal department issues the same contract to DMC members as to investigators, which usually would not have this indemnification language. Writing the contract is the responsibility of the sponsor's legal department but DeMets, Fleming, Rockhold et al. (2004) provide useful guidelines. Mutual indemnification, rather than just sponsor indemnifying DMC members, is often discussed. Most sponsors prefer just to indemnify the DMC members. It makes no sense for the DMC members to indemnify the sponsor without reciprocal indemnification of DMC members by the sponsor.

It is not uncommon for a contract research organization (CRO) to take charge of DMC operations on the part of the sponsor. In signing contracts for DMC service, members should be cognizant of what entity they are contracting with. If contracting with the CRO there is no problem in agreeing to mutual indemnification with the CRO. However, the CRO agreement will not cover DMC-member indemnification from the sponsor. In these cases, a separate agreement with the sponsor will be needed.

Almost all people joining DMCs want some form of indemnification. Sponsors often send out contracts to members that do not have an indemnification clause. Time is wasted as the members send the contract back for the addition of a clause and more time is wasted as that clause is further negotiated. It would be considered best practice for sponsors to always include an indemnification clause in the first draft of the contract.

2.8 Sponsor-DMC Relationship

The sponsor staff may be considered the "officers" of the trial and, due to their stewardship the DMC members the "board of directors" of the trial. Neither is solely responsible for the trial. In order for the DMC to be able to fulfill its role the tone must be set from the top. The sponsor sits at the top. It is their trial, their money. The sponsor must respect the responsibility and authority of the DMC and must repeatedly acknowledge that they want the DMC to do a good job and help them in protecting patient safety and trial integrity. The sponsor should not intimidate the DMC by showing emotion as DMC recommendations are read. At the same time, the DMC should not intimidate the sponsor with a "holier than thou" attitude or one of suspicion of their motives. This relationship will evolve over time. It may not get off on exactly the right foot but it is the role of all players to make this important relationship work.

Sponsor attitude will contribute much to DMC morale but the DMC has the advantage of being an ad hoc unit formed for a single purpose and never to come together in this form again. This employment strategy is known as the *"Hollywood Model."* Management experts have pointed out that teams formed in this way tend to have higher morale and are more efficient than teams of salaried employees with indefinite tenure and many see it as the future of work (Davidson 2015).

2.9 Interdisciplinary Training

While serving on a DMC, biostatisticians need to learn about the disease process, physicians need to learn about statistical methods used, and both need to learn the details of the mode of action of the drug, pathways, cascades, kinetics, and so on. The DMC–sponsor relationship should be one of continuous on-the-job interdisciplinary training.

2.10 In Conclusion

We now have learned about the within-sponsor and outside-sponsor members of the safety monitoring team and their roles. In the next chapter, we will see how these players interact in meetings.

DMCounselor

Q2.1 I am a physician chairing a DMC for an Infant Pharma. The trial my DMC has been working on is about to come before an FDA advisory committee as a pivotal trial and I have been asked by the sponsor to present the efficacy results at the meeting. Given that I am a member of the DMC should I be doing this?

A You have hit upon an important point. As a DMC member, you should not appear as an advocate for the product. That is for the sponsor and perhaps for other consultants. Explain to the sponsor that it is in their interest that they look for someone else. Perhaps, you can help by recommending some appropriate consultants.

Q2.2 I am a biostatistician who was asked seven months ago about serving on a DMC for a phase III trial that was about to begin. I called the sponsor several times to reaffirm my interest. Each time, I was told that DMC organization was to begin shortly. The sponsor finally sent me a contract yesterday but I have also learned that the trial began two months ago and dose adjustments have already been made due to early adverse events. Should I join this DMC?

A Unfortunately this situation is not uncommon. This is a sponsor who may feel that the DMC implementation, although a requirement, is an annoyance and has made it of low priority. This may make it difficult for the DMC to have the appropriate stewardship. If you feel that you can educate the sponsor for improvement of their DMC operations, then it might be worth joining the DMC. If not, I would turn down their offer.

Q2.3 I am a project manager for a sponsor (Infant Pharma) trying to follow our SOPs in forming a DMC for our upcoming pivotal trial. NIH is a cosponsor of this trial and they are insisting that their standing seven-person advisory committee serves as DMC for this trial. There is nobody on this committee that we would have chosen for our DMC because the members have little or no drug development experience. We fear the committee members will continue to fulfill the functions expected of them by NIH but not provide the proactive monitoring required by the pharmaceutical industry. What should we do?

A It is good to have NIH as a cosponsor and the prestige and credibility they can bring to this trial. Your company does not want to jeopardize these benefits with a dispute over the DMC. You must seek a win–win solution. How about proposing to NIH that your company will form a three-person DMC for the reasons that you have given and this DMC will make regular reports and share information with NIH's standing committee? Perhaps, the NIH committee would consider making the chairperson of the DMC an ex officio of the standing committee. It's worth a try.

Q2.4 I have been asked to serve on a DMC for a glaucoma product. The trial is a phase IIIB label extension trial. The product was approved several years ago and has been used by 100,000 patients postmarket. The sponsor wants to compare several schedules and drop certain arms at an interim analysis. However, I have learned that the trial has already begun and the sponsor will send us contracts and draft charter a few weeks before the first scheduled interim analysis. Sponsor claims there is no rush to do this paperwork because they already know a lot about the safety of this drug. The SOP for forming DMCs are in place and are followed for pivotal trials but the sponsor staff had made the decision that it is not necessary to follow the SOPs for a trial like this. Hearing this attitude has drastically reduced my enthusiasm for serving on this DMC. Am I being narrow minded about this?

A No, your concern is appropriate. There may be some question of whether or not an independent DMC is needed for this trial. However, the sponsor has made the decision that they would like an independent committee to help them with certain decisions they will face in this trial. You and your fellow members should explain to the sponsor that given that they decided that an independent DMC would be employed on the trial they should follow the same SOPs they have for pivotal trials. To have two standards is confusing for employees and their informal way of going about this can lower the standards for monitoring this trial which will result in an inferior trial from which nobody will benefit.

Q2.5 I am the biostatistician member of a DMC evaluating an experimental mood disorder drug sponsored by an Infant Pharma company. I have been working with the DAC biostatistician for six months now and I find that I am spending a lot of time teaching this person basic statistical methods. The DAC is a CRO and the biostatistician they have assigned is really more of a computer programmer than a biostatistician. I never expected to have to spend so much time on this and there is little return on the time that I spend because there are still many misunderstandings due to the lack of statistical knowledge. If I don't supervise this person, I don't know who would do so because the sponsor does not have a biostatistical staff.

A You should not be supervising the DAC biostatistician any more than you should be writing the statistical sections of the clinical trial report for the regulatory submission. It was the sponsor's responsibility to hire a qualified DAC and the DAC's responsibility to provide a qualified individual to serve as DAC statistician and to provide adequate training and supervision to this person. Your problem is that you need someone to talk to that understands your requirements. The Infant Pharma sponsor may not have a biostatistical staff but they must have biostatistical consultants. Similarly, the DAC may have senior biostatisticians on staff or as consultants on retainer. You ought to tell the sponsor that you want to now communicate with someone like this who can, in turn, communicate requirements to and check the work of the DAC biostatistician.

Q2.6 I recently agreed to serve as a biostatistical member on an allergy trial for a Middle Pharma company. The first version of the contract did not include an indemnification clause. I had to contact the sponsor representative 3–4 times before a version came with such a clause. When I read the clause, it read that I would be indemnifying the sponsor with no reciprocation. Surely the sponsor could not have thought that I contacted them repeatedly requesting an indemnification clause because I was concerned that I would not be able to indemnify them. Is this just the beginning of a comedy of errors with this sponsor?

A I can understand your surprise and frustration. You certainly did the right thing by asking for the indemnification clause. The error was likely caused when the sponsor representative sent the contract back to a paralegal who did not understand the context of the request. I would suspect that the attorney at the sponsor had a chuckle upon hearing about this mix-up. You ought to also have a good laugh over it and now proceed with the job you were recruited for.

Q2.7 I am a sponsor representative at a Big Pharma company. Our company just acquired another Big Pharma company. As a result, my colleagues and I are spending a lot of time reconstituting DMCs because physician members serving on our committee have consulting contracts with the company we are acquiring which put them over the conflict of interest dollar limit we have established. The physicians will continue to provide these consulting services but must now leave the DMCs. The vice president we report to is concerned how much time we are spending on this task. This is the third time in 4 years that an acquisition we made caused this reconstitution nightmare. He asked if we can make an exception to the conflict of interest limit when we make an acquisition under the justification that we only recruit people we can trust to the DMCs. I replied if that were true, why would we ever be concerned about conflict of interest. Can you help with this conundrum?

A I sympathize with the workload created by this acquisition. Hopefully some good will come from the larger company. One reason mergers and acquisitions in Big Pharma take a long time is because all sorts of potential conflicts must be negotiated. You are participating in a microcosm of that effort. I think it best to follow the SOPs regarding conflict of interest defined by dollar amount cutoffs. Surely the workload cannot be used as a dispensation. Should a company that makes a Big Pharma merger once every 50 years be required to follow the conflict of interest SOPs while one that makes three mergers in 4 years be relieved of this responsibility?

Q2.8 I am an academic gastroenterologist and I have served in the past on an FDA advisory committee. I did not enjoy this responsibility. The meetings are too long, there is too much preparation, and I didn't get a chance to speak as much as I would like due to some long-winded speeches by fellow committee members. I have now been asked to serve on a DMC. Would I like DMC service or is my experience with the advisory committee predictive of disappointment on a DMC?

A The DMC responsibilities are 180 degrees from the FDA advisory committee. I think you feel you are better at one-on-one discussions than proceedings that resemble a congressional hearing. The typical DMC consists of two physicians and a biostatistician. The meetings are with a relatively small group of sponsor representatives and you will have ample time to present your views. It is almost like one-on-one consulting. Also, it is not likely that any member will make long speeches. People like that require large audiences and video cameras.

3

Meetings

PREVIEW   The DMC Charter is a guideline for DMC scope, organization, and operations. The orientation meeting between the sponsor staff, DMC, and DAC will establish the ground rules for DMC operations and communications. The sponsor and DMC Chair will chair this meeting jointly. All subsequent meetings will be chaired solely by the DMC Chair. The data review meetings will have an open session with sponsor staff DMC members and DAC biostatistician present followed by a closed session with the DMC members and the DAC biostatistician present. The Data Review Plan (DRP) will guide DMC data review.

KEY WORDS: *DMC Charter, Data Review Plan (DRP), open session, closed session, investigator brochure, protocol, informed consent, SAE data flow, integrated summary of safety, risk evaluation and mitigation strategy (REMS), minority enrollment*

3.1 DMC Charter

We have now learned about the purpose and formation of a DMC. Before turning to the structure of DMC meetings, it is important to describe the *DMC Charter*. The charter is prepared by the sponsor and, as a result of SOPs, is very similar for all trials conducted by the sponsor except for trial-specific information. The charter will serve as a guide to meetings as well as the topics of the remaining chapters of this book. Table 3.1 lists the contents of a typical DMC Charter.

3.2 Types of Meetings

Many DMC meetings are a blend of several of the meeting types presented here. Some meetings are face-to-face and some are by telephone. The orientation meeting should be face-to-face. No face-to-face meetings should be held on sponsor's premises. Doing so can reduce the feeling of independence

TABLE 3.1

Items Typically Found in a DMC Charter

---

1. Formal name of clinical trial
2. Membership
3. Requirements for conflict of interest and confidentiality
4. DMC responsibilities
   a. Safety monitoring
   b. Efficacy data—interim analyses
   c. Publications
   d. Confidentiality
5. Chairperson responsibilities
6. Sponsor responsibilities and contact information
   a. Who is unmasked within sponsor, CRO?
   b. Who does the DMC report to?
7. Masking policy for DMC members
8. Data Analysis Center responsibilities and contact information
9. Communication and data flow between DMC, sponsor, and DAC
10. Software validation requirements, extent of data monitored at
    clinical sites before data review meetings
11. DMC recommendations
12. DMC meetings
    a. Types of meetings
    b. Schedule of meetings
    c. Open and closed sessions
    d. Voting
    e. Masking policy
13. Procedures for recommending major changes to the protocol
14. Resignation/termination of DMC member and replacement
15. Meeting minutes and retention policy
16. Safety analysis plan—templates of tables and listings to be reviewed
    during DMC meetings

---

between the DMC and the sponsor. There have been attempts to hold face-to-face meetings while DMC members are attending annual medical meetings such as the American Society for Clinical Oncology or the American Academy of Ophthalmology. In practice, many sponsors now avoid scheduling face-to-face DMC meetings at these annual congresses because of many time conflicts among members, some of which do not arise until the member arrives at the meeting.

3.2.1 Orientation or Organizational Meeting

This is the kickoff meeting where all of the players involved in DMC operations come together to review the DMC Charter and the *Safety Monitoring Plan* (SMP). The SMP might be called a PSAP (Program Safety Analysis Plan) or a DRP (Data Review Plan). There are some distinctions between these and we will explain those as we go along. The DMC members will have reviewed the DMC Charter, protocol, and investigator brochure prior to this meeting. It is highly advisable that this meeting be face-to-face.

3.2.2 Data Review

The *data review meetings* are those scheduled meetings where the sponsor will bring the DMC members up to date on trial operations and the DMC members will have a closed meeting to review the safety data.

3.2.3 Ad Hoc

As the term implies, the ad hoc meetings are called for a specific purpose usually to address a safety concern.

In the next section, we describe the nature of these meetings in detail.

3.3 Orientation Meeting

3.3.1 Chair for Orientation Meeting

Generally, the sponsor will have appointed a member of the DMC to serve as Chair prior to this meeting. Leaving the Chairpersonship up to an election among members is not advisable. The sponsor must select a person whom their staff can work with and who can do the job expected. The Chair and the sponsor representative will usually co-chair the orientation meeting. All future meetings, regardless of attendees or location, will be chaired solely by the DMC Chair. This is necessary to preserve the independence of the DMC.

3.3.2 Introduction of the Safety Monitoring Team

The sponsor representative will introduce all sponsor staff involved in the trial, as well as the DMC members and the DAC staff. The sponsor staff will usually consist of the study manager, others from clinical operations, and internal safety monitoring committee sometimes referred to as pharmaco-vigilance, firewall, or medical governance committee.

3.3.3 Appointment of DMC Secretary

The *DMC Secretary* can be a member of the DMC or the DAC statistician. It is not uncommon for the DAC to assign a project manager to sit in on closed sessions with the DAC statistician. When a project manager is present this person would serve as secretary. The secretary will prepare the minutes of each closed session meeting and circulate for approval. Only DMC and DAC members will receive copies of the closed meeting minutes.

A plan for records retention should be made at this meeting. The records must be stored in a place where sponsor staff associated with the trial will not have access until the trial is completed.

3.3.4 Presentation of DMC Charter

The co-chairs will carefully go over the DMC Charter accepting comments and revisions throughout the meeting. The typical sections of a Charter are presented in Table 3.1. We will be going through the items in the Charter throughout this book. The Charter represents the guidelines for operations and responsibilities of the DMC.

3.3.5 Masking Policy

An important decision to be made at the orientation meeting is the policy of masking which will be an item in the Charter. The Charter should indicate who at the sponsor can be unmasked. This should not be members of the sponsor's trial team but perhaps people in a pharmacovigilence group. It is important for the DMC members to know who can be unmasked at the sponsor because of important discussions of serious adverse events that may need to take place during the trial. While Middle Pharma and Big Pharma sponsors will usually have a pharmacovigilence group, this will not routinely be the case for Infant Pharma. If no such group exists the sponsor must supply the name and contact information of a consultant who would be unmasked and capable of making the types of decisions necessary if contacted by the DMC. The Charter will also indicate if the DMC will be unmasked to treatment assignment or partially unmasked. For the latter, the members know the treatments only as A or B. There is much controversy on this matter but it is agreed that DMCs may vote in closed session to be unmasked at any time. Those who advocate partially masked DMCs argue that there is no reason for anyone involved in the trial to be unmasked until absolutely necessary.

Many DMC members feel they can better understand the safety issues if they know which patients are in the experimental group and which are in the control or placebo group. These members feel that if they were selected because they could be trusted with the stewardship of the trial, why should they not be trusted with knowing the identity of the treatment groups. Indeed, many persons serving on DMCs consider it unethical for them to be masked to treatment identity. In many trials, DMC members can usually guess which treatment group is experimental after a few data review meetings due to the observed pattern of adverse events. However, there is always the chance that they might guess wrong and, if so, this can upset decision making down the line.

All documents issued during the trial that list sponsor, CRO, and DMC members should clearly indicate, usually with an asterisk, those members who are unmasked. This will minimize the chance that an unmasked person will accidentally unmask a person who is to remain masked. The usual unmasked people are the DMC members, the DAC biostatistician, and the DAC project manager if there is one.

3.3.6 Investigator Brochure

The sponsor representative will lead a summary of relevant sections of the *investigator brochure*. This document summarizes all data known about the compound under investigation. It will include safety and pharmacological data from animal studies as well as from earlier clinical trials. The investigator brochure will usually also include safety information on molecularly similar compounds. This document will suggest to the DMC members what safety issues to be on the alert for during the trial. At the conclusion of the investigator brochure discussion, there should be agreement between sponsor staff and DMC members of what adverse events are expected and what events expected to be rare are nevertheless of interest.

In this era of rapid drug development, sponsors will often begin phase III trials with fewer exploratory trials completed than had been the case in the past. This is definitely, but not exclusively, the case in Infant Pharma. This deficit in exploratory trials often prompts concern among DMC members about the dose and schedule being employed in the phase III trial. There is a definite impact of a sparse investigator brochure on the mindset of DMC members and the safety monitoring procedures they will recommend. At one extreme, members may be more likely to terminate a trial due to toxicity in this case. At the other extreme, they may operate more conservatively than otherwise especially if the drug is not in a class of drugs with similar molecular structure on which they can presume a safety profile.

3.3.7 Protocol

The sponsor representative will lead a discussion of the *protocol*. Here, DMC members will be interested in eligibility requirements, the frequency of visits and evaluations, dosing and schedule, planned interim analyses, adverse event grading and coding conventions to be used, and so on. The DMC may recommend changes in eligibility, dose, and schedule during the trial. Given the safety profile of the drug, the DMC members may recommend additional and/or more frequent diagnostic testing during the trial of procedures such as stress echocardiography, sophisticated pain scales such as the McGill Pain Index (Melzack and Torgerson 1971), or the Hamilton Depression Scale (Hamilton 1960). DMC members often want clarification about whether patients assigned to the control group will be allowed to crossover to the experimental treatment after they exit the trial if they wish and, if so, will there be continued data collection on them. When multiregional trials involve developing countries, members with clinical trial experience in these countries may want to inquire about how patient follow-up, patient compliance, SAE definitions, and so on, will be implemented and monitored in these countries. Minority under-enrollment in clinical trials has been a long-standing problem (Gorelik, Harris, Burnett et al. 1998; Heiat, Gross, and Krumholz 2002; Murthy, Krumholz, and Gross 2004;

Ford, Howerton, Lai et al. 2008; Powell, Fleming, Walker-McGill et al. 2008; Schneider, Swearingen, Schulman et al. 2009; Lechleiter 2014). Many believe that a factor in lack of clinical trial participation by African-Americans is a general suspicion of clinical trials stemming from the Tuskegee Syphilis Experiment (Caplan 1992). Hence, it is not unusual for DMC members to inquire what plans, if any, exist to ensure minority enrollment in the trial and how will this be monitored throughout the trial.

3.3.8 Informed Consent

Informed consent agreements are written by the institutions and approved by their IRBs. Sponsors usually provide a suggested wording providing their knowledge of expected adverse events. Most often, DMC members will give their input on the contents of the sponsor's suggested wording at the orientation meeting. This wording will be revisited as safety issues arise during the trial.

3.3.9 Data Flow

An important aspect of the orientation meeting is a discussion of data flow between the sponsor and DAC and the DAC and the DMC. The first item of discussion is the schedule for sponsor sending DAC the data needed to fill the tables and graphs requested by the DMC. The second item would be the schedule of the DAC sending tables, listings, and graphs to the DMC prior to a meeting. The third item would be communication of serious adverse events (SAEs) to the committee. We will define this important regulatory/clinical term in Chapter 4 but, as the term suggests, it is an event worthy of DMC scrutiny. Table 3.2 presents a checklist for issues to be decided for this

TABLE 3.2

Issues for Discussion at Orientation Meeting on Serious Adverse Event Data Flow

1. What information will be in the report?
2. Who at the sponsor will be responsible for communicating SAEs to the DMC?
3. Which SAEs will be reported—all, only those possibly related, and unexpected?
4. Will SAEs occurring on other trials not within the jurisdiction of this DMC be reported to the DMC? By whom? With what frequency?
5. Will the DMC review all deaths, only those related, and only those occurring early in treatment? How will this review be handled?
6. SAEs occurring at any time or only those occurring within 90 days of administration of study drug?
7. Will notification be as the requested SAEs occur or cumulative by week or month?
8. Will the SAE notifications first be sent to the DMC Chair and the Chair will decide what further action is needed or will all DMC members receive the SAE reports at the same time?
9. Will communication of SAEs be via e-mail? If so, this e-mail should be password protected.
10. How often will these SAE reports be updated as new information arrives?

important communication. It should be noted that the orientation meeting is the beginning of a dialog between the DMC and the sponsor on data flow requirements. It is not expected that all decisions will be finalized at this meeting.

This meeting will, at least, begin a dialog between the DMC and DAC on statistical methods to be used in reports. Table 5.8 presents a list designed to help in this discussion. At the time the DAC begins implementation of the statistical methods into their computer programming, they should issue a Statistical Analysis Plan (SAP) to the sponsor and DMC for approval and further comment.

3.3.10 Useful Software

Many sponsors and DACs are now using Internet-based enterprise collaboration software to support DMC communication. This software allows DMC members to share information over the Internet. All documents needed by the DMC such as the investigator brochure, protocol, charter, SAE reports, tables, listings, and graphs are posted at a secure website. Members are alerted by e-mail when new information has been deposited. This communication method saves paper and, since DMC members don't carry hard copies of documents, the chance of leaving a confidential document somewhere is reduced. This approach is rapidly becoming standard. When software of this type is to be used, a demonstration of its use at the orientation meeting is recommended. If a member prefers to receive documents by another means, such as paper reports sent via express mail carrier, this request will usually be granted.

3.3.11 Review of Integrated Summary of Safety

It must be decided at the beginning of the trial if the DMC will have responsibility for review of the *integrated summary of safety* (ISS). The latter is a compilation of safety data across trials in the clinical program. This document is created as part of the regulatory submission for marketing approval. DMC members will want to be sure that safety issues that they raised in their review of the confirmatory trial are not lost when the data are combined with smaller trials that may have had different patient eligibility requirements, doses and schedules, and so on. Fairweather (1996) and Weihrauch and Kubler (2002) provide useful insight into the structure and use of the ISS. The sponsor may not want the DMC to review the ISS because it may be created some time after the DMC's final meeting and the trial team may not want the DMC to get on the critical path countdown to submission for fear of slowing down the process. Whether or not the DMC reviews the ISS may be a matter of discussion at the orientation meeting. The final decision on this responsibility must be made clear at the time of the forming of the DMC.

3.3.12 Policy on Review of Publications and Package Inserts

If the DMC will have the responsibility for reviewing manuscripts on the trial that contain data reviewed by and decisions made by the DMC, this responsibility should be clarified at the meeting. A means for adjudicating disagreements on the contents of the manuscript should be formulated. Some DMCs request the right to submit their own manuscript or letter to the journal when there is disagreement. It is hoped that the latter will not have to be used but some experienced DMC members feel that this is necessary in the event that sponsors underreport adverse events in publications. DMC review of manuscripts would be considered important to ensure that there is adequate reporting of incidence and severity of adverse events and reasons for discontinuation. Ioannidis and Lau (2002) provide useful guidelines for adequate reporting. It should be noted that it might not be practical for DMC members to review the final manuscript before submission because it will generally be prepared long after the DMC has disbanded and the sponsor staff will have likely moved on to other responsibilities or even other employment by the time it is finalized. However, it is possible for the DMC to reach agreement with the sponsor on what safety issues should appear in the final manuscript at the time of their last meeting.

Closely related to the review of manuscripts would be the DMC's review of *package insert*. Although the DMC can comment on the sponsor's proposed package insert, the precise wording must be negotiated with the regulatory agencies, which have the final say.

Some regulatory agencies, such as the FDA, require sponsors to create *risk evaluation and mitigation strategies* (REMS) and *Elements to Assure Safe Use* (ETASU). For adverse events of concern, these regulations require that sponsors specify that prescribers receive special training before being able to prescribe the drug, that the drug be administered only in certain settings, patient education on warning signs of onset of events, liver function monitoring while the patient is taking the drug, and so on. If DMCs find an adverse event that lends itself to an REMS or ETASU, they certainly may raise this concern with the sponsor (U.S. Food and Drug Administration 2015c).

3.3.13 Data Review Plan

The Data Review Plan (DRP) will consist of tables, listings, graphs, statistical methods, adverse event coding conventions, and so on, that will be presented to DMC members at the periodic data review meetings. Some sponsors refer to this document as the *Statistical Analysis Plan* (SAP). However, the SAP is an important document indicating the details of the interim and final statistical analyses of efficacy and safety and is beyond the scope of the DMC. To avoid confusion we prefer the term DRP. More recently sponsors have been creating a *Program Safety Analysis Plan* (PSAP) (Crowe, Xia, Berlin et al. 2009) but this document is an important roadmap for the final safety analysis in a clinical program. In the next chapter, we will see that the DRP will be an important subset of the SAP and PSAP that relates to DMC activities.

At the orientation meeting, the sponsor and DAC will present the mock tables, listings, and graphs that they are planning to prepare for DMC review. The DMC members will provide their own ideas. This is the beginning of a dialog but a schedule for finalization should be agreed upon at the meeting. The following chapters will describe useful data summaries and statistical methods. At the end of the remaining chapters, we will introduce a table indicating the items from that chapter that might be included in a DRP. A cumulative list will be found in Appendix Table A.2.

3.3.14 Schedule First Data Review Meeting

The last item for an orientation meeting would usually be scheduling the first *data review meeting*. It is common to schedule a meeting after X patients have been enrolled or after X patients have been enrolled and completed Y cycles of treatment. However, it is important that a maximum time for first data review be scheduled in case enrollment is slow due to recruitment problems or more than expected patients being not eligible. This is done so that early enrolled patients are not unduly at risk for lack of data review just because enrollment is slow. A better wording for first meeting schedule would be "after X patients have been enrolled and completed Y cycles of treatment or after Z months whichever occurs first." A plan must also be made of the frequency of subsequent data review meetings. The plan will be a moving target depending on enrollment and data flow issues but some plan should be put in place at the organizational meeting. It should be observed that the frequency of meetings will decrease when there are fewer patients still under treatment.

Table 3.3 summarizes some of the agreements to be made at the DMC orientation meeting.

3.4 Data Review Meetings

As a general rule, there should be at least one face-to-face data review meeting each year. The others can often be handled by conference call but face-to-face data review meetings may be more frequent depending on the complexity of the trial and developing issues. There are usually a total of 2–3 data review meetings each year but the frequency will depend on the specifics of a given clinical trial. At the time a data review meeting begins, the sponsor will have a copy of tables, listings, and graphs of safety items with all treatments pooled while DMC members will have a copy with data presented by the treatment group. The latter may be presented in coded form. Data review meetings consist of *open* and *closed* sessions.

TABLE 3.3

Agreements to Be Made and/or Discussions Started at the DMC Orientation Meeting

1. Designation of DMC Chair if not previously decided
2. SAE data flow (Table 3.2)
3. Who will prepare minutes of the open and closed sessions and where will they be archived?
4. Modifications to the protocol, case report forms, and informed consent
5. Suggestions on Data Review Plan (DRP) content, e.g., adverse events of special interest, format of tables, listings, and graphs for data review meetings
6. DMC preferences for statistical methods in the DRP
7. Will Internet software be used to distribute data review materials to DMC members?
8. Masking policy for DMC members, sponsor staff
9. What unmasked group or individual does DMC report to on routine basis, when serious safety concerns emerge?
10. Plans for data quality control and software validation for data used for data review meetings
11. Will the DMC review publications, package insert, and integrated summary of safety?
12. Will data quality at sites be monitored entirely by site visits or will centralized statistical monitoring be used?
13. Budget issues for DMC operations
14. Will the DMC be briefed on final results of the trial?
15. Will data review meetings be held in person or by telephone/WebEx?
16. Description of other committees such as endpoint adjudication committee and steering committee and their relationship
17. Schedule for first data review meeting

3.4.1 Attendance

The entire safety monitoring team will be present for the meeting—sponsor staff, DAC statistical representative, and DMC members. The DMC Chair will run the meeting and the DMC Secretary will record minutes. Certain parts of the meeting will be considered open and others will be closed to all but DMC members and the DAC statistician.

3.4.2 Open Session

3.4.2.1 Study Progress

The Chair will open the meeting making sure that the minutes of the previous meeting have been accepted and then call on the sponsor representative to make a report of study progress. Before beginning the report, the sponsor representative will ask the DMC members if anything has changed since the previous meeting that might affect conflict of interest. If a member indicates in the affirmative, further discussion between this person and the sponsor will take place outside the meeting. The report of study progress will consist of enrollment progress, number of active investigator sites, adverse events of note for all treatment groups pooled, and so on. This will also be a time for the sponsor to call protocol amendments, informed consent changes, investigator brochure updates to the attention of the DMC, and ask for advice and approval. The sponsor representative will also report on the progress of tasks initiated by the DMC at previous meetings.

3.4.2.2 Data Quality

It is understood that, at the time of a data review meeting, site monitoring will not have been performed to the extent for a completed trial but the sponsor should report on the approximate percentage of adverse event data, laboratory values, and so on, that have been site monitored. A key part of this presentation would be the distribution of the last date of contact for data to be reviewed in the closed session. This will provide some idea of the currency of the data. If an SAE is under investigation and there have been, say seven cases reported, but the last dates of contact range from 3 to 6 months previous, the DMC might want an updated analysis sooner than at their next scheduled meeting.

At this point, DMC members will generally comment on any problems with the tables, listings, and graphs that they received in advance of the meeting. DMC members must be careful to speak only in general terms and not reveal trial data. This agenda item of the open session will close with the DAC statistician providing written certification that the computer programs used to generate the tables, listings, and graphs for the meeting have been validated according to industry standards. A list of standards employed by the DAC would be useful. Glaser (2002) has provided some insight on quality criteria for statistical programming.

3.4.2.3 Update on Pending Action Items

The Chair will then ask for a report of sponsor progress on issues brought up by the DMC at previous meetings. This may mean getting clarification on measurements from the central laboratory, writing a "Dear Investigator" letter, investigation of noncompliance, and so on.

3.4.2.4 Questions for the DMC

Many sponsors prefer to close the open session with specific questions that they want the DMC to take up in their closed session. The DMC may, and usually will, take up additional issues of their own choosing. Typical sponsor questions would be "Is there concern about the hypersensitivity reactions?", "Is there any concern about mortality?", and "Can the trial continue without protocol modification?"

3.4.2.5 Sample Agenda for Open Sessions

Experience has found agendas for open sessions that are merely lists of topics and do not clearly indicate responsibilities, the preparation needed, decisions to be made, and so on, that have been found insufficient. An example of a useful format is displayed in Table 3.4.

3.4.3 Closed Sessions

At the closed session, the DMC will meet together with the DAC statistician and go over the tables, listings, and graphs that were produced for the meeting. The DAC statistician will generally submit a data summary report to the DMC a short time before the meeting. It is best for DMC members to read this report *after* reviewing the meeting materials themselves. This is recommended to preserve the independence of the DMC and to ensure that members review material using the specific expertise for which they were appointed. It is useful for the DAC statistician's report to include a summary of pending safety issues.

Members will review pending safety issues and seek evidence of new issues. The precise procedures to be followed will be described in the following chapters. The DMC has the right to hold an executive session in which all DAC members would have to leave the room for the duration of the executive session. At the conclusion of the closed meeting, the Chair will contact the sponsor representative to give a verbal overview of the meeting and indicate when the minutes of the open session will be available for review. The open session minutes will be prepared by sponsor staff or CRO staff. They should follow the agenda for the open session such as the sample agenda in Table 3.4.

3.4.4 DMC Meetings for Open Label Trials

Some clinical trials are open label. Certainly single-arm trials such as those for mechanical heart valves (Grunkenmeier, Jin, and Starr 2006) are open label. Nevertheless, a DMC is advisable for independent review of safety. The format of these meetings is an open session in which the sponsor staff and the DMC discuss the safety parameters. This is followed by a closed session that enables the DMC members to discuss the implications of the safety profile among themselves.

3.4.5 Scheduling of Next Meeting

The next meeting will be scheduled in accordance with the frequency indicated in the charter unless a meeting is needed sooner to respond to a safety issue or to get a briefing from a consultant with expertise outside of the realm of the DMC members. When the next regular data review meeting is scheduled, the DAC representative will indicate a cutoff date for accumulated data that will be necessary for the DAC staff to prepare tables in time for the meeting.

TABLE 3.4

Sample Agenda for a DMC Open Session

Date: February 26, 2016

Place: Chicago Airport Hotel, Chicago, IL

Attending: Sponsor P.T., R.F. [T], L.R. T.Z, J.C.

    DMC: C.L.*, R.A.*, V.L.*, S.R.*

    CRO: A.Q.* [T], M.B.

    [T] By telephone, *Unmasked

Telephone and WebEx Info: 855-555-9745 sponsor.webex.com

Meeting Objectives: Updates on study progress

    Updates on outstanding issues

    Sponsor informs DMC of specific questions they would like addressed

Preparation: Review minutes of the last meeting—Group

    Create update reports, cutoff date 02/12/2016—T.Z.

    Review draft "Dear Investigator" letter—Group

    Research compliance situation among Latin American sites—A.Q.

    Create monitoring report, cutoff date 02/12/2016—A.Q.

    Create DAC report—M.B.

    Provide tables, listings, graphs, etc., as required by DRP to DMC for discussion in closed session—M.B.

    Checklist of changes to reports agreed to at the last meeting—M.B.

    Create a list of questions for DMC—P.T.

Decisions to be made: Is enrollment satisfactory—DMC

    Approval of "Dear Investigator" letter—DMC

    Has Latin American sites compliance improved—DMC

    Changes to safety reports completed—DMC

    Monitoring, software validation sufficient—DMC

    Plans for the next meeting—Group

(Continued)

TABLE 3.4 (*Continued*)

Sample Agenda for a DMC Open Session

Item	Time	Discussion Leader	Preparation	Decisions/Actions	By Whom	By Date
Attendance	09:00	C.L.				
Minutes of last meetings	09:05	P.T., C.L.	P.T.—Send minutes of the last open meeting for review, C.L.—Comment on approval and retention of closed meeting minutes	Approval of open meeting minutes	Group	02/26/2016
Trial status report	09:10	T.Z.	Obtain latest registration information by site, cutoff date 02/12/2016	Has enrollment improved? Additional sites needed?	Group	02/26/2016
Deaths and discontinuations due to study drug	09:30	T.Z.	Obtain pooled data cutoff 02/12/2016	Discussion in closed session	DMC	
Draft "Dear Investigator" letter	09:45	J.C.	Write the draft and circulate to DMC members no later than 02/19/2016	Discuss wording and send out	DMC	Mail final version by 03/03/2016
Compliance report Latin America	10:00	A.Q.	Obtain update on compliance in run-in meds at Latin American sites	Has there been improvement? Further action needed?	DMC	02/26/2016

(*Continued*)

TABLE 3.4 (*Continued*)

Sample Agenda for a DMC Open Session

	Time	Person	Description	QUESTIONS		Date
Cardiac event adjudication review	10:15	A.Q., J.C.	From adjudication meeting 12/03/2015	QUESTIONS	DMC	02/26/2016
Protocol deviations	10:30	A.Q.	From internal meetings	APPROVAL	DMC	02/26/2016
Charter and protocol amendments	10:45	A.Q., J.C.	From internal and DMC discussions	Approval	DMC	02/26/2016
Status of changes in reports requested by DMC at the last meeting	11:30	M.B.	Use list of changes requested by DMC issued 10/31/2015	Have requests been satisfied?	DMC	02/26/2016
Status of software validation	11:30	M.B.	Obtain status of validation of software used for generation of tables at this meeting	Is this level adequate?	DMC	02/26/2016
Questions for DMC in closed session	11:35	P.T.	Meet with staff to draft list prior to 02/26/2016			
Closed session	11:45–13:30	C.L.				
Open session—Debriefing	13:45	C.L.				
Plans for the next meeting	14:15	C.L., P.T.		Sponsor staff to make arrangements	P.T.	03/07/2016

3.4.6 Minutes

Two versions of the *meeting minutes* will be issued. One will cover the open session and be distributed to sponsor staff. This version should clearly describe sponsor, DMC, and DAC responsibilities for the next meeting together with deadlines. The DMC version will cover both the open and closed sessions and include a list of pending safety issues that will need to be revisited until resolved.

3.5 Ad Hoc Meetings

The DMC may need to schedule ad hoc *meetings* to deal with emerging safety issues. These meetings will usually be run by conference call and will be closed session only. The agenda for the ad hoc meeting will be similar to that for the data review meeting. This meeting may be held without sponsor's knowledge but, if with sponsor's knowledge, the sponsor would usually not be informed of the agenda for the meeting.

3.6 In Conclusion

This chapter has introduced the types and organization of DMC meetings. In our next chapter, we will investigate the nature of the clinical data that the DMC reviews.

Table 3.5 presents a list of some DRP items that are approved and/or created before the start of the trial. Table 3.6 displays a list of potential DMC

TABLE 3.5

Items for Inclusion in the Data Review Plan (DRP)

Details of SAE data flow
Expected patient accrual graph, expected rate of screen failures
Goals for enrollment of minority patients
Method of transmitting data review materials to DMC members
Unmasked sponsor group or individual DMC contacts when safety concern arises
Will site monitoring or centralized statistical monitoring be used?
Estimated time from data cutoff to DMC meeting
Data review meeting frequency
Frequency of face-to-face meetings
Use of telephone/WebEx for meetings

Note: A complete list of DRP items appears in Appendix Table A.2.

TABLE 3.6

Potential DMC Responsibilities Arising in This Chapter

Comment on and approve charter

Comment on and approve initial Data Review Plan (DRP)

Comment on protocol and investigator brochure

Comment on informed consent form and subsequent changes

Comment on and suggest changes to SAE data flow

Clarify the role of DMC in

Design of integrated summary of safety

Manuscripts/publications

Risk evaluation and mitigation strategies (REMS)

Package insert

Make sure the relationship among the DMC, Steering Committee, Internal Safety Review Committee, and Safety Assessment Committee is understood by all

Note: A complete list of DMC responsibilities will be found in Appendix Table A.31.

responsibilities arising in this chapter. A complete list of DRP items and DMC responsibilities will be found in Appendix Tables A.2 and A.3, respectively.

DMCounselor

Q3.1 I am a DMC Chair. The sponsor just sent me and each of the DMC members an e-mail indicating that they are postponing our data review meeting scheduled for three weeks from now. They claim that the DAC has not had time to do the programming to prepare for the meeting. We don't want to postpone the meeting and we took a considerable amount of time to get our calendars in order for the scheduled meeting. Do we have to comply with the sponsor's change of date?

A The first issue is that the sponsor has no right to change the date of a DMC meeting. The DMC sets the dates and only the DMC can change the date. The sponsor should have contacted you, the Chair, alone and tried to get your input on what could be done. The second issue is that the DAC should be more responsive to the requests of the DMC. There is usually more than enough time to do the programming between meetings. You may have no choice but to postpone your meeting but this would be a good opportunity to have a heart-to-heart talk to get the sponsor–DMC–DAC relationship on the right track.

Q3.2 I am a physician member of a DMC for a randomized active control trial in seasonal allergic rhinitis. The active control is a marketed drug for this indication. The tables we review show that there is a consistent 18% incidence of transient headache which we can confidently attribute to the experimental drug because we know that this does not occur at all on the active control. I am in favor of terminating the trial because I am confident that no physician is going to prescribe a drug with this side effect when the active control and other marketed drugs do not have this side effect. My fellow DMC members think that such an extreme action would be out of line. What should we do?

A   The issue you raise is a marketing issue and not a serious safety issue. The DMC is not charged with making marketing decisions and it is not clear what the marketing potential will be once the efficacy data are known. Your concern is understandable but, for now, just concentrate on the serious adverse events. At the end of the trial, I am sure the sponsor will value your input on marketing issues like the one you raise.

Q3.3   I am an oncologist serving on a DMC for an oncology trial sponsored by an Infant Pharma company. At our open meetings, the sponsor representatives take a lot of time asking the DMC members advice on matters that do not concern patient safety. Many of the questions have to do with what licensing opportunities the company might pursue with Big Pharma and if the company should be writing protocols to show the combined efficacy with a popular kinase inhibitor to increase licensing potential with that company. I do not feel comfortable or qualified to answer these questions but our Chair and one other clinician member seem eager to discuss these matters. How do we get back on course?

A   It appears that you have uncovered an important agenda item for your closed meeting. The DMC members are not contracted to provide such advice and it is thus out of scope. The Chair is obviously not running the open session as he/she should be. If so, this type of questioning should not take place. At your closed session, you should just remind the Chair that these business topics are not appropriate DMC issues and try to build consensus to politely deflect these kinds of questions should they appear again.

Q3.4   I am the biostatistical member for a DMC working on an experimental drug used in emergency medicine. All clinics participating are emergency rooms. The other members of the committee are all ER physicians. We have had two telephone data review meetings so far and a face-to-face meeting is now scheduled for 5 months hence. The members are very competent in emergency medicine but as we look at the very nice safety tables produced by our DAC, our Chair will interrupt with questions about waiver of consent and selection bias and the other members will begin giving their experiences with these issues. I have heard some of their experiences more than once even in the same meeting. As time passes, beepers go off, we run out of time, and I feel the meeting adjourns with not enough time spent reviewing the safety tables. How do I move this committee in the right direction?

A The good news is that the ER doctors on your committee definitely understand the concepts of doing clinical trials in emergency rooms. There are certain standards upon which informed consent can be waived due to the emergency nature of the encounter and, indeed, selection bias can occur because the most severe patients may be treated off-protocol with approved medicine immediately because there is not time to go through the enrollment and randomization process. However, there is no reason to be so obsessed with these issues that the DMC's safety responsibilities are compromised. It would be sufficient for the DMC Chair to ask the sponsor team at each meeting if waiver of consent is being followed and if the sponsor's monitors have any evidence of patients who would be protocol eligible being treated off-protocol. These are really sponsor responsibilities and not direct DMC responsibilities. You should diplomatically remind your Chair of this and also use your DMC's Charter to show that these issues do not fit neatly into a DMC responsibility category. There is no problem in asking the sponsor for clarification of this matter should there be disagreement with your interpretation. However, there is no doubt that independent safety review is critical. It is possible that the physicians on your DMC might have looked at the safety data prior to the meeting, decided there was nothing serious to discuss, and were thus comfortable curtailing the meetings. This, of course, is not acceptable and the minutes of your meetings should note that the safety data were not discussed in detail. You might want to request a "catch up" safety review by telephone rather than wait 5 months for the next meeting.

Q3.5 I am a biostatistician serving as Chair of a DMC for an antiulcer drug. The trial also has a steering committee. The DMC unmasked from the start of the trial, the sponsor and steering committee members unmask along with investigators after all patients have completed 16 weeks of treatment. The trial continues until all patients have completed 52 weeks of treatment. The unmasking point is about to take place and the sponsor has called a first-ever joint DMC–steering committee meeting. At the meeting, the sponsor wants the DMC to hand over its responsibilities to the steering committee for the rest of the trial under the justification that everyone will now be unmasked, the steering committee will have definite continuing responsibilities so that they might as well take over the review of safety data after the DMC briefs everybody on safety issues to date. Needless to say, this sudden announcement has decreased the morale of the DMC. We feel we are the safety experts for this trial, we are independent of sponsor, and we have a fiducial responsibility to continue to operate until the end of the trial. How do we solve this?

A It appears that this problem has arisen because the sponsor made this decision a few days before they called this meeting. The change of safety responsibility was not a documented procedure before the trial began and the surprise would not be expected to go over well with the DMC members. Sponsors do not like to work with multiple committees but we must give them credit for supporting at least two committees during the masked phase. At the unmasking, the sponsor would probably like to reduce their workload and expense by just dealing with one committee. As you say, everyone is unmasked and the steering committee members probably have similar credentials to the DMC members. However, I agree that the DMC members have the trial memory and reached their decisions while masked. A reasonable compromise might be for the steering committee to meet periodically with you as an ex officio member. At the end of the trial, there can be another joint meeting with the DMC. This seems to be a compromise that takes advantage of the DMC expertise but also is not an unreasonable overkill of advisors for the unmasked phase.

Q3.6 I am a neurologist and Chair of a DMC working with Big Pharma on an Alzheimer's disease treatment. We scheduled a data review meeting and three weeks before the date of the meeting, the sponsor told us that our meeting must be postponed. The reason for the postponement was that our meeting would occur 2 days before the sponsor's quarterly report to shareholders. If there were something negative in our meeting, they would have to report it publicly in the quarterly report. They acted like surely we would understand and agree to the postponement. I was furious with this statement. The DMC is supposed to be independent of the sponsor. We are supposed to do our work regardless of the consequences for the sponsor. Eventually, the sponsor representative got back to us and said that management decided that since we had set the date before they had made this policy, our committee would be grandfathered and we could meet on the date decided. I am not sure this was a victory.

A There are many constraints in the setting of a meeting date but this is the most self-serving I have ever heard. It is an affront to the very purpose of a DMC. You have every right to be upset. Yes, your meeting will now proceed as planned but, in the future, your DMC will propose meeting dates and the sponsor might just say "not good for us." They will certainly not reveal the reason if it is quarterly report time. There is much in the sponsor–DMC relationship that we have not worked out and we will see more emerging issues in Chapter 8. For now, you should lead your committee in the careful monitoring of patient safety regardless of what day the sponsor's quarterly report is due.

Q3.7 I am an African-American cardiologist now serving on a DMC for a hypertension product for a Big Pharma sponsor. This is the third Big Pharma sponsor that I have served as a DMC member. The pattern that keeps repeating is that when I bring up enrollment in the trials, various philosophical discussions begin as to the cause and concern with low minority enrollment. They indicate that my suggestions are excellent but I am not sure they are carried out and I have not seen an improvement. How can I be more effective?

A You deserve a lot of credit for what you are trying to do and the sponsors you have worked with should realize that they can benefit from more diversity in enrollment. The fact is the sponsor staff is under intense pressure to enroll patients. They have some skill in motivating investigators to improve enrollment and in bringing more sites into the trial when enrollment is lagging. The sponsor staff does not have the skills to deal with a problem as complicated as minority enrollment. I would advise you to suggest to these sponsors that they hire a minority enrollment "czar" who can work with sponsor staff across trials, keeping score, trying various approaches, and so on. This is the sponsor staff person that you want to interact with. It is only with this kind of specialist input that we can hope to make progress.

Q3.8 I am Chair of a DMC working with a privately held Infant Pharma sponsor on a pediatric epilepsy product. My DMC members and I understand that it will likely be impractical for us to review the final manuscript for this trial. However, we know the trial terminated 6 months ago and we haven't heard from the sponsor since our final data review meeting. Should we not be debriefed by the sponsor on the final results of this trial, at least as a courtesy?

A Unfortunately, this omission happens with privately held companies more frequently than it should. The investigators are debriefed when the trial ends and there is no apparent reason why the DMC members cannot be included in that communication. As we have listed in Table 3.3 above, this is a matter that should be discussed and agreed upon at the DMC orientation meeting.

Q3.9 I am the biostatistical member of a DMC working on a pain medication for a Big Pharma sponsor. At the orientation meeting, the sponsor described the secure web portal that will be used to send us data review materials. However, they neglected to tell us that user passwords expire every 3 days. This means that we have to change passwords at least twice during our data review meeting preparation. In addition, if we need help with using the system, we must communicate with the sponsor's IT department. All the DMC members are based in the United States but our IT contact is in Germany. This gives a narrow window of time when we can contact him and most of us do our DMC data review work in the evening because we have day jobs. Evening in the United States corresponds to the middle of the night in Germany. Even when we call him during day hours in Germany, we can only get help from him when he is available. We have complained to the sponsor staff about all of this but they just tell us it is out of their hands. The IT department is assigned to provide this support, not them.

A This situation is untenable. Without sufficient changes from the sponsor, they will have to revert to sending members paper reports or reports on password-protected CDs. The sponsor must understand that IT procedures that might apply to their employees are impractical for DMC members. Passwords should not change with the frequency you report. Also, employees of the sponsor are not dependent on one person in Germany. They can always get help from a non-IT person in the office next door to them or from an on-site IT person. If Internet data distribution is to continue, a DMC IT plan will be needed and it will have to include 24/7 support.

Q3.10 I am Chair of a DMC working on a treatment for advanced breast cancer. Our meetings are administered by a CRO. We have a five-member committee. At our last meeting, one of our members did not phone in at the appointed time and the CRO project member just said "OK we have a quorum let's get started." The project manager did not seem to care that this person was not present. What would be the best practice here?

A The most important issue here is that you, the Chair, of the DMC, must run both the open and closed sessions of data review meetings and NOT the CRO project manager. This is necessary for independence. You are the one to decide when to proceed if a member has not yet called in. Also, since the open session precedes the closed session, there is time for you, the Chair, to assign someone on the sponsor staff to try to contact the missing member and, at least, have that person on the line for the closed session. For future meetings, be sure to tell the CRO project manager that you are chairing both open and closed sessions.

Q3.11 I am Chair of a DMC for an Infant Pharma sponsor. From the first meeting, I have asked the sponsor's medical director for a contact person outside the company to serve as a pharmacovigilance consultant should the DMC have a serious safety concern. This has gone on for three meetings now and she has not produced a name. What can I do to get this moving?

A It is unfortunate that you have not gotten a name from the medical director this much into the trial. You need to explain to her that, should there be a safety concern, you would not want to ask her at that point for the name of a consultant because that would signal that a problem exists and it might even lead to some unmasking at the sponsor. Hence, if you do not receive the name of a consultant, the DMC would have no choice but to stop the trial. This should get her attention. To be fair, she may have been looking for a consultant and been turned down either because her candidates have conflicts of interest or it is a responsibility with too much pressure for a person who has little knowledge of the compound in the trial. If this is the case she should explain this to you. Perhaps, you can talk to your fellow members for names of people who might serve and present those names to the medical director for consideration. If she has several candidates, there is no reason why the DMC cannot interview candidates and help her with the decision.

Q3.12 I am Chair of a DMC working on a rheumatoid arthritis treatment for an Infant Pharma sponsor. Instead of giving us a Data Review Plan especially prepared for the DMC, they have asked us to read through their Statistical Analysis Plan for the entire trial. Our biostatistical member is spending a lot of time making comments on analysis methods, bias, regulatory agency preferences, and so on, that have nothing to do with the scope of our DMC. I have told her that she should be selective of her comments but she insists what she is saying is important and the sponsor needs to hear her comments. What should I do to get us back on track?

A First, your DMC should be proud to have such a qualified and motivated biostatistician as a DMC member. The sponsor should have prepared a DRP at the beginning of the trial and then the biostatistical member would not have seen out-of-scope details in the first place. It is still a good idea that this be done and perhaps you and the biostatistical member could work with the sponsor staff on such a document. The biostatistical member should just advise the sponsor that they need to retain qualified statistical support for their SAP and that she is not the right person for this task.

Q3.13 I am Chair of a DMC for a pediatric solid tumor trial. We have retained a renowned pediatric hematologist to be a voting member of the committee due to our concerns of neutropenia as an adverse event. With this person's advice, we advised the sponsor to make dose adjustments in the protocol. We left the meeting proud of our decision but one week later, the sponsor told us that the steering committee overruled our decision. We were never told that the steering committee would review our decisions or had the authority to overrule. The steering committee consists of senior oncologists but they do not have anyone who knows as much about neutropenia as our member. How do we straighten this out?

A   This confrontation is what sponsors and DMC Chairs fear when more than one committee is involved. Of course, this dispute would have been avoided had the relationship between committees been clearly established at the outset. The DMC always reports directly to the sponsor on matters of safety and interim analysis of efficacy. There is no precedent of the hierarchy you describe and there is always the suspicion that the steering committee was called in only because the DMC recommended dose adjustment. However, the DMC recommendation for dose adjustment is only advisory to the sponsor. The sponsor can overrule this and can seek the help of others in making this decision including members of the steering committee. This does not mean that the steering committee has an official role here to review DMC decisions. The sponsor can be faulted for telling you that the steering committee overruled. The representative could have just justified the sponsor's decision not to adjust dose at this time without any reference to what person or persons may have given input.

Q3.14   I am a biostatistician serving on a DMC for an infectious disease drug. This is my first DMC experience and so far I am enjoying it and feel that I am contributing. The only problem is that I have mentioned several things that I think the DMC should take up such as an advertising campaign to increase enrollment in the Asian clinical sites, making contact with a DMC working for the same sponsor on the same drug for a different infectious disease to compare notes, and so on. Each time, the Chair says that he must check our charter to see if we are allowed to do these things. When he looks, he will come back and say that he did not see my items specifically listed and therefore they must be considered out of scope. This sounds like a U.S. Supreme Court justice reading the constitution. Am I guilty of being overzealous in this new endeavor? Is the charter supposed to be read so strictly? Are we not here "to provide for the general welfare"?

A   You are to be complemented for your enthusiasm and for the new ideas you bring. I am sorry that your Chair is reading the charter in that manner. One problem often stated about charters is that they are too long and detailed which leads to the problem you have encountered. You ought to tell your Chair that the charter, just like the U.S. Constitution, is meant to be a general guideline and cannot possibly list all of the tasks that a given DMC might see fit. I might also say the two ideas you had are right on. Suggesting strategies for increasing enrollment and sharing safety data in the way you describe are definitely areas the DMC should involve itself.

Q3.15   I am the biostatistical DMC member for a Big Pharma sponsor on a vaccine trial in the developing world. There are five pediatric virology experts serving with me on the DMC. They have all known the sponsor staff for some time. I have learned a lot from these people and really enjoyed the experience. I use the past tense because the trial ended and we were debriefed in a detailed conference call. The sponsor is continuing to schedule meetings to go over marketing strategies and potential postmarket protocols. It is nice to be invited to these meetings but I feel that I contracted only for the trial and do not feel that I can be that useful in this extension. I want to end this engagement but I do not want to burn any bridges and don't want them to think that I am ungrateful for the opportunity they gave me. How do I handle this?

A I agree with your assessment of the new situation. You should not feel guilty. I am sure the Charter for this DMC did not include this extension. The committee is no longer a DMC but rather a post-market strategy consulting group. You might explain to the sponsor that you do not feel that you would be of value for this new committee. The sponsor is likely to agree with you but did not want to alienate you by being the only member not invited to continue.

4

Clinical Issues

PREVIEW The primary goal of DMC safety review is to separate signal from noise. Regulatory agencies have recently issued guidance documents asking sponsors to evaluate risk versus benefit and asked them to make assessments of experimental drug causality of serious adverse events. These directives have an effect on DMC responsibilities. The sponsor's responsibility in reporting SUSARs (Serious Unexpected Suspected Adverse Reactions) should involve DMC communication. MedDRA is the standard adverse event dictionary in industry-sponsored trials. Adverse event severity is graded by WHO or CTCAE criteria. Multiregional trials require extra scrutiny due to social, political, and demographic differences.

KEY WORDS: *adverse event severity, adverse events of special interest (AESIs), adverse event tiers, CTCAE, Final Rule, granularity, MedDRA, multiregional trials, pharmacovigilence group, standardized MedDRA queries (SMQs), SUSAR (Serious Unexpected Suspected Adverse Reaction)*

4.1 Goals of Safety Analysis

The ultimate goal of safety analysis in clinical trials is to describe and evaluate patient risk for treatment-emergent adverse events. To accomplish this, DMC members must separate adverse events that are part of the disease process, preexisting or concurrent conditions, and those that are related to a concomitant medication from those that are related to study drug. In short, safety analysis seeks to separate signal from noise. To accomplish this goal, DMC members will review tables and will occasionally use methods of statistical inference but discussions of possibly serious treatment-emergent adverse events will not be solely dependent on the result of a statistical hypothesis test. Statistical methods appropriate for DMC safety analyses will be covered in Chapter 5.

The past decade has seen an increase in an attempt to standardize safety reporting and analysis in clinical trials. This effort has come from governmental groups, international organizations, and industry groups. The recent trend has been prompted by interest in consideration of safety in terms of *risk versus benefit*. The U.S. FDA has issued guidances on premarket risk assessment (U.S. Food and Drug Administration 2004b), risk minimization action plans (U.S. Food and Drug Administration 2005), safety assessment for investigational new drug (IND) safety reporting (U.S. Food and Drug Administration 2015a), risk evaluation and mitigation strategies (U.S. Food and Drug Administration 2015b), safety data collection in late-stage development programs (U.S. Food and Drug Administration 2016), and what has become known as the *"Final Rule"* on expedited safety reporting (U.S. Food and Drug Administration 2012). CIOMS Working Group IX has also issued recommendations for risk minimization (Council for International Organizations of Medical Sciences 2015).

The ICH has issued E2F on the development safety update report (International Conference on Harmonisation 2010) and E2C on periodic benefit–risk reports (International Conference on Harmonisation 2012) and the European Commission has issued CT-3, the detailed guidance on the collection, verification, and presentation of adverse event/reaction reports (European Commission 2011). In addition, a pharmaceutical industry group known as *SPERT*—Safety Planning, Evaluation, and Reporting Team—has issued guidelines for developing detailed safety analysis planning prior to the start of confirmatory trials (Crowe, Xia, Berlin et al. 2009; Xia, Crowe, Schriver et al. 2011). Another pharmaceutical industry group—Benefit Risk Action Team (*BRAT*) has issued a framework for benefit–risk assessment (Levitan, Andrews, Gilsenan et al. 2011). These new guidelines apply mostly to sponsor safety analyses and operations. However, some have implications for additional DMC responsibilities in safety monitoring and will be covered in this chapter and in Chapter 5. These guidance documents have much overlap, so, it will be difficult to cite precisely where the ideas or recommendations that follow originated. The latter are also cited in various review papers, which will be cited in what follows. The FDA also issued a guidance on *risk-based monitoring* (U.S. Food and Drug Administration 2013). This will be discussed in Chapter 8.

4.2 Definitions

Safety analysis entails continuous surveillance of many variables with many subclassifications in the effort to look for signals of risk. The need for common definitions and terminology in drug safety is a long-standing problem (Meyboom, Lindquist, and Egberts 2000; Aronson and Ferner 2005), The World Health Organization (WHO) made an early attempt to standardize adverse event terminology (Edwards and Biriell 1994) as did the Council for International Organizations of Medical Sciences (CIOMS) (Venulet and Bankowski 1998). ICH has published harmonized definitions for use in clinical trials for investigational drugs in their E2A guideline (International Collaboration on Harmonisation 1994). The following definitions are paraphrased from E2A.

4.2.1 Adverse Event

An *adverse event* is any unfavorable and unintended sign (e.g., including an abnormal laboratory finding), symptom, or disease temporally associated with the use of a drug, whether or not considered related to the drug. The term *treatment-emergent* is often added as a modifier in order to remove manifestations of preexisting conditions from consideration.

4.2.2 Serious Adverse Event

A *serious adverse event* (SAE) is any untoward medical occurrence that, at any dose, results in death, is life-threatening, requires inpatient hospitalization or prolongation of existing hospitalization, results in persistent or significant disability/incapacity, or is a congenital anomaly/birth defect.

An important distinction is between a *severe* adverse event and an SAE. Severe refers to the intensity of the event but not necessarily to the seriousness. A patient may experience a severe headache but it would not be considered serious by the above definition. Similarly, a mild case of dehydration might cause hospitalization and thus be considered serious. It is helpful to remember that an SAE is a regulatory/clinical term while severe adverse event is completely a clinical term. We will explore shortly how severity of adverse events might be defined.

4.2.3 Adverse Event Tiers

The SPERT (Crowe, Xia, Berlin et al. 2009) recommended that adverse events be divided into three tiers. *Tier 1* is a list of AEs for which specific hypotheses and analysis methods are described before the trial begins. These would be adverse events suggested by preclinical studies, early phase clinical trials, and/or knowledge of the drug class. *Tier 2* consists of AEs that were not prespecified but have become apparent in safety monitoring in this trial and where there are a sufficient number of events for data analysis. SPERT has recommended that an AE type that is not in Tier 1 that has been observed with at least 1% frequency in any treatment group automatically qualifies that AE type as a Tier 2 event (also cited in Chuang-Stein and Xia 2013). *Tier 3* events are infrequent events that do not lend themselves to statistical analysis but will be presented in listings. Adverse events are not often presented to DMCs in terms of tiers but DMC members should be aware of this classification and work with sponsors to create this trichotomy as the trial progresses.

4.2.4 Serious Adverse Event Reporting Requirements

Regulatory agencies require expedited reporting of SAEs when they are unexpected. The latter would mean that there are no previous documented cases of this SAE for this drug either in the literature or in the investigator brochure. Investigators are asked to exercise judgment on whether the SAE was unrelated, possibly related, or related to study drug. Expedited reporting requirements vary between regulatory agencies but such reporting is often required for unexpected SAEs that occur within 28 days of study drug administration or after 28 days if the investigator deemed them at least possibly related (U.S. Food and Drug Administration 1997). IRBs and DMCs will receive expedited SAE reports. All other SAEs will be reported periodically to IRBs, the DMC, and to the regulatory agency.

4.2.5 Serious Unexpected Suspected Adverse Reactions (SUSARs)

In the Final Rule (U.S. Food and Drug Administration 2012), FDA asked sponsors to make expedited reports of *SUSARs* (Serious Unexpected Suspected Adverse Reactions). The SUSAR is, in the United States, wholly a sponsor designation of an unexpected severe AE being causally related to the experimental drug. The rule was designed to reduce the number of expedited reports (7–15 days) submitted by sponsors since "causality" meets a higher test than "associated." However, this classification provides an important responsibility for DMCs to be in a continuous dialog with sponsors on what AEs should be considered SUSARs. Wittes, Crowe, Chuang-Stein et al. (2015) define three categories of serious adverse events which would qualify as final rule SUSARs—*Category A*: rare events that are usually drug related (e.g., agranulocytosis, Stevens–Johnson syndrome, and angioedema). *Category B*: adverse events not commonly associated with drug exposure but also uncommon in the patient's demographic group (e.g., myocardial infarct among young women) and *Category C*: events that occur more frequently in the experimental group than control group throughout the clinical program. This categorization might be useful to DMCs in advising sponsors of SUSAR candidates. It is important to note that an adverse event might be suspected, such as neutropenia in an oncology trial or a myocardial infarct in the older population in an Alzheimer's trial, but if it occurs at a higher rate than expected it is considered a SUSAR. Another possible complication of SUSAR interpretation is that in the United States, the SUSARs are determined by the sponsor but in Europe by the individual investigators. This will provide an analysis and regulatory challenge.

Of course for a sponsor to make a decision that a certain adverse event has been caused by the experimental drug it is necessary for the sponsor to unmask. However, the sponsor team assigned to this protocol should not unmask but rather the pharmacovigilence group mentioned previously. For Big and Middle Pharma, this should not be a problem for Category A and Category B events. Unmasking even the pharmacovigilence group for Category C events is problematic. While there is agreement that the DMC should advise on SUSAR matters, there has been no discussion of a DMC having sole responsibility for creating Category C events and, indeed, Category C may not be used by sponsors as a criterion for determining SUSARs. For Infant Pharma, the SUSAR regulation makes it imperative that they have a team of outside experts who can function as a contract pharmacovigilence group.

4.3 Safety Data

4.3.1 Pharmacovigilence Groups

Safety data will be processed at the sponsor in accordance with its SOPs and will be transferred to the DMC in accordance with the data flow plans in the DMC Charter. For Big Pharma and most of Middle Pharma, expedited serious adverse event data are processed through a separate pharmacovigilence group within the organization. This group is separate from the team working on the trial. The procedures of some sponsors allow or require this group to be unmasked to the treatment of the patient who experienced the event. Other sponsors insist on masking. In any event, the team working on the trial should be masked. For the Infant Pharma companies, there is no clear pattern but most choose for everyone in the company to be masked. This is done partly for scientific reasons but also to minimize the possibility of SAE-treatment information to leak to investors and the financial community. As was noted earlier Infant Pharma companies would be expected to identify an outside resource to handle pharmacovigilence.

4.3.2 Case Report Forms

All adverse events and laboratory values will be reported along with other clinical trial data on case report forms (CRFs). These forms will eventually be sent to the sponsor either electronically or by mail for processing for the final regulatory submission. The CRFs will record the description of the event, dates of onset and resolution, grade or severity of the event, and the relatedness to study drug. The latter is open to investigator judgment. Definitions exist for determining grade and severity of an event and these will be described below.

4.3.3 Adverse Event Dictionary

The adverse event reports must be coded in accordance with a dictionary. This is done by the sponsor's pharmacovigilence staff. The pharmaceutical standard for adverse event terminology is *MedDRA—Medical Dictionary for Regulatory Activities*. MedDRA was created in the 1990s as a joint venture between the International Federation of Pharmaceutical Manufacturers and

Associations (IFPMA) and ICH. MedDRA is available through software on a subscription basis through the Maintenance Support and Services Organization (MSSO) (MedDRA Maintenance Support and Services Organization 2016). ICH provides periodic "Points to Consider" updates on the use of MedDRA (International Collaboration on Harmonisation 2007). The MedDRA dictionary (Brown, Wood, and Wood 1999; Bousquet, Lagier, Lillo-Le Louet et al. 2005) provides a hierarchy of terms beginning with system organ class, and progressing through preferred terms, high-level terms, and so on. For example, a system organ class might be "Blood and Lymphatic System Disorders" and preferred terms within this class might include anemia, coagulopathy, eosinophilia, hypoprothrombinemia, thrombocytopenia, and so on. The number of preferred terms generated within an organ class in an adverse events table will be referred to as the *granularity* of the table. Many of the adverse events enumerated for the marketed drugs in Appendix Table A.1 represent combinations of several preferred terms. Sponsors usually follow a written internal policy for how combinations are to be made to define common adverse events such as headache, nausea, and dizziness. We will come back to granularity as a possible source of bias or inferential pitfall in Chapter 6. However, much progress has been made in the past decade in an attempt to confront granularity as an analytic issue with the development of SMQs. The SMQ is a *standardized MedDRA query*. These queries were developed by the MedDRA organization though advisory committees of clinical experts. An example of an SMQ would be MACE—a major adverse cardiac event. MACE combines MedDRA terms, all-cause mortality, myocardial infarct, and target vessel revascularization. There are other SMQs for convulsions, depression and suicide/self-injury, hypersensitivity, and many more (Chuang-Stein and Xia 2013; MedDRA 2013). In addition, many sponsors have created their own proprietary SMQs that are needed for the particular drugs and indications in their confirmatory trials. DMC members should be aware of all SMQs to be used in the trial they are serving. Schactman and Wittes (2015) discuss various strategies for combining MedDRA terms for DMC use.

In looking at Appendix Table A.1, we also note that heart blockage and bradycardia are listed as adverse events for cardiovascular drug metoprolol, angina pectoris for cardiovascular drug ramipril, and arthralgia for osteoporosis drugs risedronate and teriparatide. These were clearly adverse events observed in the trial but are also likely part of the disease process. Making these distinctions is an important role for DMCs.

4.3.4 Adverse Event Severity

It is essential that some system be used to attach a degree of severity of the adverse event. A coding system assigns an increasing AE intensity score called a *severity* or *grade*. Severity is generally coded as "none," "mild," "moderate," "severe," "life-threatening," and grade as 0, 1, 2, 3, and 4. "None" and

TABLE 4.1

Severity Score

Severity	Definition
None	Adverse event not experienced.
Mild	Transient, requires no special treatment or intervention, does not generally interfere with usual daily activities, and includes transient laboratory test alterations.
Moderate	Alleviated with simple therapeutic treatments, impacts usual daily activities, and includes laboratory test alterations indicating injury but without long-term risk.
Severe	Requires therapeutic intervention, interrupts usual daily activities.
Life-threatening	Requires significant therapeutic intervention but the patient is at *immediate* risk of death.

"0" are the codes assigned to patients who did not experience the adverse event in question. Table 4.1 presents common definitions of severity. Codes for grades are generally written for particular medical specialties using criteria based on data commonly collected in these fields. Examples are the U.S. National Cancer Institute's Common Terminology Criteria for Adverse Events (CTCAE) (U.S. National Cancer Institute 2006), the U.S. National Institute of Allergy and Infectious Disease, Division of Microbiology and Infectious Diseases (U.S. National Institute of Allergy and Infectious Disease 2007), OMERACT 7 for rheumatology (Lassere, Johnson, Boers et al. 2005), and the adverse events following immunization (AEFI) for vaccine trials (Bonhoeffer, Kohl, Chen et al. 2002).

For clinical trials in oncology, the distinction between MedDRA and CTCAE is very important. CTCAE is a dictionary intended for use by oncologists in clinical trials that they may undertake in federal government sponsored trials. MedDRA is the dictionary of choice for safety reporting by FDA and other regulatory agencies. Some pharmaceutical industry sponsors of oncology trials specify CTCAE grades to be used with MedDRA terms. Oncologists serving on DMCs may need some orientation to MedDRA if they are used to thinking in CTCAE terms. Pharmadhoc (2016) provides useful information on CTCAE and MedDRA—CTCAE mapping tools.

DMCs will most often study tables of frequency of "moderate or worse" or "severe or worse" toxicity by treatment group. This is a purely clinical determination and is considered more useful than SAE tables. The latter have the regulatory component where mild toxicity that nevertheless leads to a brief hospitalization is considered an SAE. We will return to this in Chapter 5.

4.3.5 Adverse Event Summary

Table 4.2 summarizes the various adverse event definitions described above. It is also useful to define *adverse events of special interest (AESI)*. There are

TABLE 4.2

Summary of Adverse Event Terminology

Term	Definition
Adverse event (AE)	Any unfavorable and unintended sign (e.g., including an abnormal laboratory finding), symptom, or disease temporally associated with the use of a drug, whether or not considered related to the drug.
Serious adverse event (SAE)	Any untoward medical occurrence that, at any dose, results in death, is life-threatening, requires inpatient hospitalization or prolongation of existing hospitalization, results in persistent or significant disability/incapacity, or is a congenital anomaly/birth defect.
Adverse event severity	Intensity of the adverse event as measured by a grading system such as that in Table 4.1.
Adverse Event Tiers	
Tier 1	A list of AEs for which specific hypotheses and analysis methods are described before the trial begins; adverse events of special interest.
Tier 2	AEs that were not prespecified but have become apparent in safety monitoring in this trial and where there are a sufficient number of events for data analysis.
Tier 3	Infrequent events that do not lend themselves to statistical analysis but will be presented in listings.
SUSAR	Serious Unexpected Suspected Adverse Reactions—A sponsor designation of an unexpected severe AE being causally related to the experimental drug. Expedited reporting required.
SUSAR Categories	
Category A	Rare events that are usually drug related (e.g., agranulocytosis, Stevens–Johnson syndrome, and angioedema).
Category B	AEs not commonly associated with drug exposure but also uncommon in the patient's demographic group (e.g., myocardial infarct among young women).
Category C	AEs that occur more frequently in the experimental group than control group throughout the clinical program.
MedDRA	Medical Dictionary for Regulatory Agencies—A globally popular AE dictionary.
SMQ	Standardized MedDRA queries—Define an AE type by pooling terms from several MedDRA hierarchies.

certain agreed-upon adverse event types that are always of concern regardless of drug or indication. These would include cardiac, renal, liver and bone marrow toxicity, immunogenicity, polymorphic metabolism, and the drug's abuse potential including tendency to overdose and the withdrawal effect(s). These events are discussed by Chuang-Stein and Xia (2013). They also define the AESI as being those adverse event types that sponsors should be aware of as the confirmatory trial begins. These would be adverse event types that are listed in the investigator brochure for the trial as being possibly associated with the experimental treatment or its drug class. Some DMC members may

TABLE 4.3

Clinical Information in the Data Review Plan

Data review meeting frequency—face-to-face, teleconference

Adverse event dictionary—(most likely MedDRA)

If oncology trial what will be the role of CTCAE

Standardized and proprietary MedDRA queries to be used (SMQs)

Severity-grading dictionary to be used

Sample AE narrative form (CIOMS or sponsor proprietary)

Tier 1 adverse events—adverse events of special interest

Tier 2, 3 adverse events added as trial progresses

Data flow of AEs requiring expedited reporting—see Table 3.2

Procedure for creating and updating the SUSAR list—Categories A, B, and C

Particular issues in multiregional trials

Note: See Appendix Table A.2 for a complete list of information in the Data Review Plan.

think that the AESIs should automatically become Tier 1 events discussed above. However, most sponsors do not do formal hypothesis testing for the AESIs but rather create intensified pharmacovigilence for these events.

The DRP (Data Review Plan) was introduced in Chapter 3 as being those parts of the Program Safety Analysis Plan (PSAP) and Statistical Analysis Plan (SAP) for the clinical program that apply to DMC analyses and operations. Some of the clinical content of the DRP has been defined above and is summarized in Table 4.3. A complete list of DRP items will be found in Appendix Table A.2. Statistical content will be defined in the next chapter.

4.3.6 SAE Narratives

The coding conventions described above have been created for use in generating statistical tabulations of adverse events in a manner that we will describe in the next chapter. When deaths and serious adverse events occur, physician members of DMCs want to review the narrative descriptions of the events. These descriptions are written by pharmacovigilance staff, masked to treatment assignment, after reviewing all information available including interviews with the investigator whose patient experienced the event. The narrative will describe the event by MedDRA preferred term giving patient age, gender, date of onset, investigator opinion on relatedness, medical history, relevant baseline information, comorbidities, concomitant medicines, and so on. The content of these forms is often discussed by DMC members during the closed session. These forms are also sent to regulatory agencies when the events qualify for expedited review. The narrative form is updated as new information on the event arrives. Some sponsors have their own narrative report format but the standard format used by most companies is that developed by CIOMS (Council for International Organizations of Medical Sciences 2005, 2006).

4.3.7 Titration to Dose

In some protocols, patients are titrated to dose, that is, the investigator progressively increases the dose until a dose that is "optimal" for that patient (using efficacy response and tolerability criteria) is reached. It will be important for the DMC to ascertain that the protocol for the trial provides a detailed description of how titration is performed in sequential visits, that the dose for each appears on the case report form and on SAE narratives, and that investigators are complying with the titration protocol.

4.4 Deaths

Deaths are an important consideration in DMC review. The DMC will attempt to determine if deaths are due to the disease process or to the drug and, usually, not relying solely on a comparison of treatment groups especially when an active control group is used for a life-threatening disease such as cancer. Deaths might stand out more in an allergy trial than in an oncology trial. Even in the latter, the early deaths, those occurring in the first cycle of therapy might be suspicious. Oncology DMCs use the term "death as a first event" or "death less than 30 days post treatment start" to describe this phenomenon and seek reports of these early deaths. Most DMCs will not limit their review to deaths that the investigator or sponsor pharmacovigilence unit classified as drug related. This would violate their mission of stewardship. Johann-Liang, James, Behr et al. (2005) discuss this issue in relation to deaths on HIV clinical trials. Quite a bit of judgment and second guessing is involved in these deliberations. We will return to this topic in later chapters.

4.5 Impact of Multiregional (Global) Trials

The past decade has seen an accelerating trend toward performing clinical trials globally especially in India, China, and Eastern Europe. Pivotal trials today can include investigators in Moscow or Mumbai as frequently as Memphis or Montreal. Sponsors find lower costs and higher level of trial participation in these regions than in North America. These countries have large numbers of untreated patients eager to enter trials because this is often the best route to medical care. Many investigators in these countries are Western trained, they have clinics built specifically to conduct clinical trials, they adhere to ICH guidelines, and sponsors can hire or contract with physicians (rather than nonphysicians as is the case in North America) to act as clinical research associates to monitor protocol and regulatory adherence at sites (Platonov 2003; Kahn 2006). Hence, there is motivation among sponsors to include sites in these developing countries. DMCs should be aware of varying data quality due to the lack of long experience in pharmaceutical industry trial participation and other cultural differences discussed below.

The problems encountered in multiregional trials in terms of efficacy endpoints are reviewed by Binkowitz and Ibia (2011). Regional heterogeneity in efficacy results is often difficult to explain as in the case of the MERIT-HF trial for chronic heart failure (MERIT-HF Study Group 1999), the PLATO trial for acute coronary syndromes (Wallentin, Becker, Budaj et al. 2009), and in various Alzheimer's disease trials (Luan, Muni, and Hung 2016).

The following sections review some global issues that impact the work of a DMC on safety data.

4.5.1 Cultural Issues

Geographic patterns of genetic variation have been known to affect adverse drug reactions (Wilson, Weale, Smith et al. 2001). Diets followed by some countries could interact with experimental drugs to give the appearance of drug-related AEs. Different cultures have different propensities to self-report the AEs and these personality issues are further impacted when caregivers are the chief reporters of AEs to investigators as is often the case in Alzheimer's disease and Parkinson's disease.

4.5.2 Political Issues

Some state-run European health systems present physicians with financial incentives to hospitalize patients (Haluska and Aamdal 2007). The hospitalization automatically qualifies an adverse event as an SAE. Thus, we may see more SAEs reported from these countries. DMC members should not discount SAEs being reported from any country but this is something to take into consideration. Some European regulatory agencies require sponsors to unmask whenever an SAE occurs (Stump 2007). Although FDA does not support this practice, sponsors must adhere if their trials come under these jurisdictions. Other political issues sometimes encountered would include patient attitudes due to suspicion of the capitalist system and difficulty with the concept of informed consent.

4.5.3 Medical/Surgical Practices Issues

Although Western medicine methods prevail in these new clinical trials markets, national health system formularies occasionally differ from North America in the nature of supportive care—use of anti-infective drugs, antiplatelet drugs, and so on, which can affect the level of adverse events. Similarly, funding of surgical techniques may differ and this can be a factor when study drugs are used postsurgery. For active control trials due to international differentials in approved drugs or drugs supported by national health systems the active control drug may vary over countries. Also, ethical requirements usually indicate that for certain diseases, the control group must be standard of care. However, standard of care varies between regions and DMC members may be reviewing data from trials that have varying control groups depending on investigator location.

4.5.4 Data Quality Issues

The variation of data quality (accuracy) from institution to institution is an issue even in domestic trials but becomes even more of an issue in multiregional trials. There are regional, cultural, and educational differences in the clinical staff who see patients and record data. It is important that the sponsor presents a table at each DMC meeting indicating for each country the number of active sites, number of patients enrolled, number of data queries outstanding and resolved, and the percent of source data verified to date. DMC members can make suggestions of regions where more focus may be needed. An additional issue is the quality and efficiency of translation of AE narratives to English.

Table 4.4 reviews the multiregional issues and provides suggestions for DMC investigation and response. The table mentions the possible use of logistic regression analysis. This method will be discussed in the next chapter.

4.6 In Conclusion

We have seen that there is considerable subjectivity in reporting and classifying adverse events and these factors are compounded in multiregional trials. These factors will affect a DMC's mission in separating signal from noise and in making safety decisions. There is no one perfect way to handle this situation but we will learn more about current practice in the next chapter on statistical methods.

Table 4.5 summarizes some potential DMC responsibilities from this chapter. A complete list will be found in Appendix Table A.3.

TABLE 4.4

Issues in Multiregional Trials

Issue	Possible DMC Response
Cultural	
Geographic genetic variation	Ask sponsor for literature search of what is known about genetic variation related to this disease and treatment. If this is a factor, a stratified analysis or covariate-correction through logistic regression might be requested.
Differential diets among countries	Ask sponsor for literature search of how diet might affect AE levels. If there appears to be an effect, a stratified analysis or covariate-correction through logistic regression might be requested.
Propensity to self-report AEs	Compare incidence of AEs that is self-reported between countries. If there appears to be an effect, suggest guidance to the investigators and request stratified analyses.
Political	
Financial incentives to hospitalize patients	If there appears to be a higher SAE level for an AE type in some countries than others, investigate if these are countries with financial incentives to hospitalize. If so, review the CIOMS forms to see which SAEs can be classified as AEs for DMC purposes only. If there are some perform a DMC analysis. This analysis will not be considered the official drug application analysis.
Unmasking required when SAE occurs	This should have little effect because the SAEs probably *de facto* unmask anyway.
Suspicion of the capitalist system	Investigator staff must reassure potential patients of the benefits of the clinical trial.
Difficulty with the concept of informed consent	Investigator staff members need to spend time with the patients and their families to make sure the informed consent form is well understood. Patients concerned about the potential adverse events should not be enrolled.
Medical/Surgical Practice	
Use of supportive care	Through "Dear Investigator" letter try to harmonize supportive care. When differences exist consider their impact. Stratified analysis or covariate-correction through logistic regression might be needed.
Different surgical techniques used	This may be difficult to harmonize because of differing training, skills, and equipment among countries. Stratified analysis or covariate adjustment through logistic regression may be required.
Active control may vary over countries	Perform an analysis to see if odds ratios vary for between active controls for the same AE type. If so, correction can be made through covariate adjustment in logistic regression.
Control group must be standard of care but standard of care varies among countries	Perform an analysis to see if odds ratios for the same AE type vary between countries that vary for standard of care. Correction can be made by covariate analysis in logistic regression.
Data Quality Issues	
	The sponsor should present a table at each DMC meeting indicating for each country the number of active sites, number of patients enrolled, number of data queries outstanding and resolved, and the percent of source data verified to date. DMC members can make suggestions of regions where more focus may be needed. The quality and efficiency of translation of AE narratives to English is an additional issue.

TABLE 4.5

Potential DMC Responsibilities from This Chapter

DMC members should decide on being partially masked or unmasked

Clarify Tier 1 adverse events or AESIs (adverse events of special interest)

Approve initial SUSAR (serious unexpected severe adverse reactions) list and establish the mechanism for DMC role in updating

Periodic data review following DRP (Data Review Plan) and amend as needed

Comment on

  Adverse events of concern

  Enrollment issues

  Screen failure rate

  Minority enrollment

  In multiregional trials, regional issues of concern

Note: See Appendix Table A.3 for a complete list of DMC responsibilities.

DMCounselor

Q4.1 I am an infectious disease specialist serving on a DMC for an experimental infectious disease drug. The committee agreed that we need an electrocardiologist consultant to help us interpret some of the severity of some cardiovascular SAEs. The consultant selected by the sponsor wants to hold a half-day in-service training with slides he uses to train his residents. We don't think this is necessary.

  A It sounds like the consultant believes in one-size-fits-all teaching. Although this electrocardiologist is paid by the sponsor, he/she reports to the DMC and, thus, the DMC must decide how his/her time is best spent. It is the DMC's responsibility to write out the objectives and scope of the consultant's engagement. Does the DMC really want to learn electrocardiology or do they want the electrocardiologist to look at the data on some adverse events and advise on the seriousness? It might be good for the consultant to provide some guidelines for the DMC members to judge future SAEs of this type but it might be more prudent to have the consultant return to review more cases as they develop. The key here is that the DMC must take the lead and be in charge of this not to follow what the sponsor and their favorite electrocardiologist think is right. If your DMC cannot work out an acceptable agreement with this electrocardiologist you might want to seek another consultant.

Q4.2 I am a physician and Chair of a DMC for a rheumatology indication. We have asked the sponsor for more information from some investigators on SAEs that we have been reviewing. The information has not arrived. How long should we wait before we give up?

A You are observing that DMCs operate in an imperfect world. It is the sponsor's responsibility to get this information for your committee and its representatives should be reporting to you on their progress during open sessions of your meetings. However, the sponsor too works in an imperfect world. They may not be able to get further information because such information may not exist or the investigator is just too busy to send it. If the information does not come between meetings of your DMC, you must assume that it will never come and do the best you can with the information you have while continuing to keep the request open with the sponsor until they satisfy the DMC that they have tried everything and there will be no more data.

Q4.3 The sponsor for our DMC has opted not to use a central lab for the Eastern European sites participating in this trial due to logistical problems. The North American sites are using a central lab and those in India are using a Bangalore-based branch of the North American lab. The serum chemistries coming from the Eastern European sites have a much higher incidence of abnormal values than from the other sites. These sites are not declaring the abnormal values as AEs, which is troublesome enough, but we are spending a lot of time talking about the lab values from these countries and, given that their origin is different from the other investigator sites, we are probably wasting a lot of time.

A Welcome to the world of multiregional trials. All the Eastern European sites have separate labs at their institutions. They probably have different equipment and different ways of determining the laboratory range of normal. Your DMC should review the reported AEs and SAEs of these sites carefully and ask the sponsor to find out if the patients with the abnormal values have associated symptoms that would be expected for these lab values such as neutropenia, thrombocytopenia, and liver function. You can press the sponsor for this type of clinical information because it is likely to exist.

Q4.4 I am the Chair of a DMC working on a treatment for inflammatory bowel disease. The trial began 5 months ago. To increase enrollment, the sponsor has added a Canadian site and is considering some Eastern Europe sites. The Canadian site has told the sponsor that they will not participate unless a Canadian physician is added to the DMC. My fellow DMC members and I see no need for another member and we have concern that we will soon be asked to add an Eastern Europe representative. Isn't this getting out of hand?

A The DMC must be part of any decision to add a member. However, it sounds like the sponsor has been honest with you on the reason for adding the Canadian member. Rather than resist the addition of a Canadian member, I suggest you consider the advantages of having regional representation in multiregional trials. In addition to clinical knowledge, this person brings an understanding of the practice of medicine in Canada, payment systems, regional nutritional trends, and so on, all of which could influence adverse event frequency. The DMC has a right to assess whether the candidate can provide this type of information. Eastern Europe is much different than North America and your DMC may benefit from a representative from this region if sites are to be established there. Of course, this can get out of hand if Latin American and African sites are to also be added. At that point, the sponsor might agree to add the additional members only after 6-month accrual quotas are met. If these quotas are not met, there would be less need for the additional regional members.

Q4.5 I chair a DMC for a chronic leukemia trial for an Infant Pharma sponsor. At our first data review meeting, I raised the question of why we did not receive the SUSAR current list. The sponsor surprised my fellow committee members and me by saying that the SUSAR list comes from a different database than the clinical data we review. The data we see originate with investigators while the SUSAR data are a sponsor product. I realize that SUSAR is a new concept but, given the nature of the SUSAR data, should we not be reviewing this list as a matter of course?

A Actually SUSAR is not that new a concept. It is the sponsor's opportunity to submit to regulators a shorter list of SAEs than previously and save sponsor, regulators, and DMCs some work. It is certainly not a commercial confidential proprietary list that should not be shared with the very people who are supposed to advise on product safety on the basis of accumulating data such as that displayed in the SUSAR. I certainly agree with you and your committee members. You should explain the situation to the sponsor representative and indicate that regardless of the database in which SUSAR is located as a result of the Final Rule, it is an important document for DMC review.

Q4.6 I am the biostatistical member of a DMC working with an Infant Pharma sponsor on a glioblastoma trial. We reviewed a list of countries participating in the trial and noted that the United States had 512 data queries outstanding while Russia had 46. We called this disparity to the sponsor's attention during the open session and one member of the sponsor team said that in Russia, the site monitoring is done by physicians deployed by a CRO while in the United States, it is recent college graduates sometimes with no clinical training who are sent out for site monitoring so that a lot of errors are missed and not resolved until late in the trial. A physician member of our DMC questioned this as an explanation. Do you think there is some other reason for this disparity?

A I certainly don't think this disparity should be brushed off with something based on the difference in education of the site monitors. It is entirely possible that the physician monitors in Russia might be second guessing the investigators and changing the case report from entries themselves. This, of course is a violation of good clinical practices but, unfortunately, in multiregional trials this kind of thing happens. I also don't understand why the sponsor representative is satisfied with U.S. site monitors he/she considers unqualified traveling all over the country at his/her company's expense. This does not sound like a cost-effective strategy for ensuring data quality. In any case, you and your committee members are correct. The discrepancy is a matter for further investigation.

5

Statistical Issues

PREVIEW We will cover numerous methods of statistical analysis in this chapter but it is important to remember that no DMC safety decision is made solely on the basis of a statistical calculation. There may be statistical significance for an AE type that is not of clinical significance and vice versa. Safety analysis should be performed on the intent-to-treat population. Statistical methods for treatment differences in AE frequency that take drug exposure into account (Poisson rate ratio, Kaplan–Meier) are preferable to those that do not (relative risk, odds ratio). Repeated tests of significance lead to the problem of multiplicity which can be controlled through the use of the false discovery rate. We introduce likelihood and Bayesian methods as alternatives to frequentist methods of statistical analysis. These methods are not yet common in DMC data review.

KEY WORDS: *intent-to-treat, screen failure rate, confidence interval, Poisson rate ratio, Kaplan-Meier, landmark estimate, relative risk, odds ratio, Type I error, Type II error, significance level, power, multiplicity, false discovery rate*

5.1 Goals of Statistical Analysis

The objective of this chapter is to review some common methods of statistical analysis that would be of use to DMCs and to demonstrate their interpretation in the context of DMC operations. Some novel methods that are of particular use to DMCs are presented. This chapter is not meant to be a statistical textbook. Thus, we will not reproduce formulas that are easily available elsewhere and/or where calculations are commonly made by readily available statistical software. Details are provided in a nonrigorous manner for certain techniques that are not as well known and may be especially of interest to the biostatistician reader.

The ultimate goal of safety analysis in clinical trials is to describe and evaluate patient risk for treatment-emergent adverse events. To accomplish this, DMC members must separate adverse events that are part of the disease process, preexisting or concurrent conditions, and those that are related to a concomitant medication from those that are related to study drug. In short, safety analysis seeks to separate signal from noise. To accomplish this goal, DMC members will review tables and will occasionally use methods of statistical inference. Unlike efficacy analysis of primary endpoints, inference will not hinge on the statistical computation of a single endpoint. Safety analysis entails continuous surveillance of many variables with many subclassifications. There will be numerous important discussions of possibly serious treatment-emergent adverse events regardless of the result of a statistical hypothesis test. The role of the DMC biostatistician will be to remind physician members of the weight of evidence while taking uncertainty into account. These are among the concepts we will discuss in this chapter.

5.2 Useful Data Displays

This section will describe certain types of tables, listings, and graphs that have been useful in DMC data review meetings. Specialized tables may be needed depending on the indication. For any DMC, the data displays reviewed should be considered a work in progress—consideration of modification should be continuous in order to properly support emerging issues and certain displays may be discontinued because they are deemed to be no longer necessary.

The DAC will prepare two versions of each table, listing and graph. One version, which will be for use by the sponsor, will have all treatments pooled. The other, for DMC use, will be presented by treatment coded as A, B, and C; Blue, Green, and Yellow; or Tulips, Roses, and Orchids. This presentation is known as *partially masked*. If the DMC is to be unmasked, a partially masked table will still be presented with the independent statistician decoding during the closed session. Partial masking is necessary in case the tables are inadvertently left in a hotel or airport lobby. More will be said about masking policy in Chapter 7. For partially masked tables, the treatment codes should be consistently matched with actual treatments at each meeting of the DMC, that is, A, B, C, and so on, should represent the same treatment at each meeting.

It is assumed that all data displays will be performed for the *intent-to-treat* population of patients meaning all patients randomized regardless of how much treatment they received during the trial. In some cases, it may make sense for analysis to also concentrate on the *adherers-only* subset being those patients who received treatment according to the protocol or some other criterion (Piantadosi 2005).

Table 5.1 presents a list of useful data displays. Note that the first two displays listed deal with patient enrollment. These are for open-session discussion and would not generally be produced on a treatment group basis.

TABLE 5.1

Useful Data Displays

---

1. Patient enrollment by center, ethnicity, and stage of disease (not usually produced by treatment group)
2. Demographic description of study cohort
3. Cumulative patient enrollment by month (not usually produced by treatment group)
4. Cumulative distribution of patient exposure
5. Table of reason for discontinuation
6. Data currency table—Data management cutoff date for this meeting, most recent death, and SAE by center
7. Treatment-emergent adverse events by body system, possibly subclassified by
   a. Grade
   b. Relatedness to study drug
   c. Event types within body system
8. Same as #7 for serious adverse events
9. Laboratory values of interest. List by patient and flag those outside of normal range
10. Amit graph of relative risks (see Section 5.8)

Note: Sponsor version for both treatments pooled, DMC version by coded treatment group.

An exception would be if there was a need to consider whether or not randomization was flawed (unbalanced by treatment group). The following is a description of each display.

5.2.1 Enrollment by Center, Ethnicity, and Stage of Disease

A listing of enrollment by center including a calculation of enrollment/ month of center participation is useful. For trials that have a *run-in screening phase* where patients qualify for randomization (see, e.g., Faught et al. 1993 in epilepsy and Thijs et al. 1995 in hypertension) this should be calculated for both phases. DMC members may comment on nonperforming sites but also, in multiregional trials, get an idea of what part of the world the patients are coming from. The DMC will comment when the *screen failure rate* is high. This is a challenge to the efficiency of the trial and, depending on the disease, there may be some strategies that could minimize screen failure rate. As mentioned in Chapter 3, there is concern about underrepresentation of minorities in clinical trials and DMC members should review the ethnicity distribution at each meeting and suggest improvements. In a life-threatening disease such as cancer, a protocol might be open for stage III and IV patients. DMC members should review enrollment by stage. It is not infrequent that DMC members note that enrollment is heavily weighted toward very sick stage IV patients. Sponsors especially worry that, although they have confidence in the efficacy of the experimental treatment, it might not perform well against an active control drug for this cohort. DMC members might suggest ways of recruiting more stage III patients or modifying the eligibility requirements for the trial to create a more favorable patient profile.

5.2.2 Graph of Cumulative Patient Enrollment by Month

This graph (example Figure 5.1) will show the total patient enrollment by months since the start of the trial. Some sponsors prefer to add the monthly estimated patient enrollment (usually a straight line) to the graph. This will enable DMC members to review enrollment progress over time. For trials having screening or run-in phases a line can be added for the qualifying phase. The estimated patient enrollment trajectory will not always be a straight line. The estimated enrollment will take different shapes if patients must experience a relapse on a previous trial in order to qualify for enrollment, in infectious disease trials where there is seasonal variation in incidence of the disease under investigation, or where the sponsor plans to phase in sites over time.

Some Data Analysis Centers (DACs) have developed sophisticated simulation methods to predict enrollment over time. These methods are a departure from typical linear projections in that they use the exponential distribution with a varying parameter over time and make adjustments to this simulation as the trial progresses. This is a valuable tool especially when there is a planned interim analysis.

5.2.3 Graph of Cumulative Patient Exposure to a Study Drug

As DMC members discuss adverse events in closed session, it is important for them to know how much exposure patients have had to the drug. If there is concern for cardiac toxicity, for example, inspection of this graph may show that since only 20% of patients have received three cycles of the drug, it is too early to dismiss cardiac events as a concern. If later in the trial, after

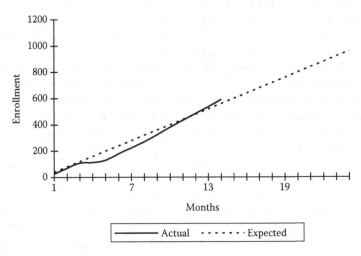

FIGURE 5.1
Cumulative patient enrollment by months since the start of the trial.

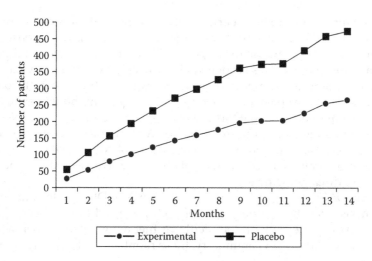

FIGURE 5.2
Cumulative patient exposure by treatment group and month since treatment start.

70% of patients have received three cycles of the drug and only 2% of patients reported cardiac toxicity, DMC members may begin to feel confident that cardiac toxicity will not be an issue. An example of a cumulative patient exposure graph is shown in Figure 5.2.

5.2.4 Treatment-Emergent Adverse Events

5.2.4.1 Classification

There are many ways to classify and analyze adverse events. The art of classification has been discussed in Chapter 4 and classification, as a source of bias will be covered in Chapter 6. For now, we will concentrate on body system, subclassification within body system, relatedness to study drug, and grade or severity. An investigator's conclusion about relatedness to study drug is a regulatory requirement. In order to be conservative, many DMCs ignore this variable in analysis especially in open label trials. The first line of any AE tabulation should be the summation of AEs for all body systems combined. This will give DMC members a sense of the number of patients experiencing AEs of any kind.

For each treatment group, the number of patients and the total exposure for the group should be presented. Exposure will often be patient years of follow-up but in some trials, the number of cycles or number of injections might be considered more relevant to safety.

Now, the table proceeds to list adverse event types by body system and the preferred term within body system. At the start of a trial, the degree of granularity of preferred terms within body system should represent the DAC's best guess of an appropriate level. The DMC can request revisions in the preferred terms after some experience accrues and will certainly review the SMQs discussed in Chapter 4. They could recommend that the sponsor considers other SMQs available through MedDRA. The art, science, and potential biases of granularity selection will be discussed further in Chapter 6. It is by no means an unimportant issue. For each AE type when the patient experienced several episodes of the same AE, the patient should generally be presented only once classified as the most severe episode. Most tables will have columns indicating the frequency of AEs by grade or severity. DMC members may prefer to consider only incidence of AEs classified as grade 3 or greater generally defined as moderate or worse. This would be especially true in life-threatening diseases.

Several DACs are now beginning to place MedDRA code numbers in parenthesis after the text definition of each preferred term. This is a good practice. As experience with the MedDRA hierarchy begins to pervade the physician–biostatistician community, these numbers will be useful to DMC members.

At any DMC meeting, the DMC may recommend changes to data displays going forward. These changes may include more information on emerging adverse events of interest and/or reducing the size and scope of data displays based on what has been learned up to that point.

5.2.4.2 Example: The APPROVe Trial

We will illustrate several analytic techniques with the example of cardiovascular events associated with rofecoxib as presented in Bresalier, Sandler, Quan et al. (2005). This trial was commonly known as the APPROVe trial (Adenomatous Polyp Prevention on Vioxx). Some controversy exists for this trial and several papers were published after the original providing correction to some data. We use the original data because it is being presented solely for illustration and not to present a point of view regarding the safety of rofecoxib.

Table 5.2 presents the data on adjudicated (confirmed) thrombotic adverse events from APPROVe that we will use in the following sections. The primary objective of the trial was to determine the effect of 3-year treatment with rofexocib on the risk of recurrent neoplastic polyps.

TABLE 5.2

Adjudicated Thrombotic Adverse Events in the APPROVe Trial

	Rofecoxib	Placebo
n	1287	1299
Patient years	3059	3327
No. of events	46	26
Incidence (%)	3.57	2.00
Rate/100 patient years	1.50	0.78

The trial randomized 2586 patients with a history of colorectal adenomous polyps to either rofecoxib or placebo—1287 to rofecoxib and 1299 to placebo. Rofecoxib patients contributed 3059 patient years and placebo patients 3327.

5.2.4.3 Incidence Calculation

The incidence calculation is merely the percent of patients in each treatment group who had experienced an adverse event—for rofecoxib 3.57% (46/1287) and placebo 2.00% (26/1299). We call the proportion of patients who experience the AE *proportional incidence*. For rofecoxib, proportional incidence is 0.0357 (46/1287) and for placebo (0.0200). It is important to note that in all safety calculations, each patient is counted only once. If there were repeat episodes of the same AE type for a patient, the patient is counted in the numerator in an incidence calculation only once.

5.2.4.4 Incidence and Exposure Time Calculation

The overall incidence by treatment group calculation would be appropriate if patients in each of the treatment groups had equal exposure to study drug. This will not be the case when there is a differential in dropout rates between treatment groups. The difference might be due to toxicity so it is important to take exposure into account.

Exposure time and incidence can be combined in either of two ways. The first is to calculate the incidence per unit time such as the number of events per 100 patient years. The second is a graphical method discussed in the next section. The rate per unit time calculation is made by dividing the number of events by the total number of patient years on the trial and multiplying by 100. In our example, the rate/100 patient years for rofecoxib is 1.50/100 patient years $(46 \times 100)/3059$ and for placebo it is 0.78/100 patient years $(26 \times 100)/3327$.

The question arises if events should be counted after the patient has experienced the first occurrence of a certain AE type and if repeat episodes of this event should be counted. The most common convention is to count patient exposure as long as the patient remains on the protocol. To do otherwise would present different numbers of patient years for each AE type and there appears to be no benefit from doing this. At some point, the DMC may want to concentrate on a certain AE type and then it may be appropriate to ask the DAC to compute rates using exposure only up to the first occurrence of that AE type. However, as we will see below, the Poisson distribution (Rosner 2006) is the reference probability distribution used for statistical inference of the rate/100 patient years and this distribution would, theoretically, require all occurrences and all exposure time to be counted in the numerator and denominator, respectively. This convention is not generally followed in pharmaceutical trials but it is standard in adverse event analysis of clinical trials of mechanical heart valves (Grunkenmeier, Johnson, and Naftel 1994).

First occurrence and exposure are more accurately computed in the following section.

5.2.4.5 Kaplan–Meier Time to First Occurrence

Kaplan–Meier time-to-event curves, which provide a graphical view of the occurrence of events over time, take the number of patients at risk at each time point into account by dropping patients who discontinue or experience the event along the way. For patients who do not experience the event, their "time to event" is just their time on study (their total time) and this observation is called *incomplete* or *censored*. Those patients who do experience the event have their time to event recorded. Their observation is called *complete* or *uncensored*. The *Kaplan–Meier* methodology, formally known as the *product limit method*, is often applied to efficacy analysis but can easily be applied to safety data. In oncology trials, the method is frequently applied to survival analysis (time to death). However, a patient can die only once but can experience the same type of adverse event more than once. We use the Kaplan–Meier analysis for adverse event data to describe the *time to first occurrence* of the event. The methodology for calculating a Kaplan–Meier curve is beyond the scope of this book but details can be found in numerous references and software is readily available (Kaplan and Meier 1958; Piantadosi 2005; Cleves, Gould, Guttierrez et al. 2008; SAS Institute 2008). Figure 5.3 displays the Kaplan–Meier curve for time to adjudicated thrombotic adverse events in APPROVe. The vertical axis indicates the cumulative number of thrombotic events and the horizontal axis indicates time. This graph suggests that the thrombotic AE experience is about

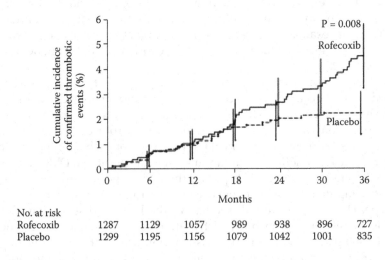

No. at risk						
Rofecoxib	1287	1129	1057	989	938	896	727
Placebo	1299	1195	1156	1079	1042	1001	835

FIGURE 5.3

Kaplan–Meier estimates of the cumulative incidence of adjudicated thrombotic events (the vertical line indicates 95% confidence intervals). (From Bresalier, R.S., *New Engl. J. Med.*, 352, 1092–1102, 2005.)

equal in both groups but that the curves begin to diverge after 18 months with more events accumulating for rofecoxib than placebo.

Kaplan–Meier time-to-event curves would not normally be routinely generated for all adverse event types. This would create voluminous output. These curves would be requested by the DMC for AE types of particular interest and usually to study the development of these events over time.

5.2.4.6 Incidence at a Time Point after Treatment Start: Landmark Estimate

It is not uncommon for DMCs to request a *landmark estimate* of incidence (sometimes referred to as a point *estimate*) from a Kaplan–Meier life table. This estimate consists of specifying the Kaplan–Meier estimate of AE incidence at a particular time point such as 12 months after treatment start. This is an estimate of cumulative incidence from treatment start up to and including 12-month posttreatment start. The estimates and their standard errors are found on listings of the Kaplan–Meier *life table* (Kaplan and Meier 1958; Rosner 2006; Cleves, Gould, Guttierrez et al. 2008; SAS Institute 2008). They can also be read from a Kaplan–Meier graph. From Figure 5.3, we see that in the APPROVe trial, both treatments have a 12-month incidence of serious thrombotic events of about 1%. This type of analysis is useful to show that certain AE types occur mostly in the first, say, 6 months after treatment start and then level off. It is important that landmark estimates of incidence be made using Kaplan–Meier methods. Computing the raw percentage of patients who experienced an adverse event within the first, say, 12 months of treatment has an obvious numerator but the denominator is difficult to compute because of patients who are censored before 12 months.

Before leaving this introduction to the Kaplan–Meier method, we should describe the *reverse Kaplan–Meier* estimate. This method is not used for efficacy (survival time) or safety (time to first occurrence of AE) but rather as a way of evaluating the degree and efficiency of follow-up in a clinical trial. Schemper and Smith (1996) recommended computing a Kaplan–Meier curve with patients who died coded as censored and those who were still alive at last contact as uncensored. The resulting median follow-up time is not penalized due to patients who died and who, thus, could not be followed up further. This method of estimating follow-up appears often in reports of oncology trials (e.g., Mayer, Van Cutsem, Falcone et al. 2015). DMC members may be presented reverse Kaplan–Meier follow-up time estimates during sponsor presentations in open session.

5.2.4.7 Other Ways of Looking at Incidence

After viewing some SAEs, it is possible that DMC members may feel that the SAEs are related to a dosing of the drug. In these cases, DMCs might request an additional table of SAEs that occurred within a time window (such as 30 days) postinjection.

We will use the term *covariate* to mean a variable that might influence AE incidence. In most cases, raw incidence rates will be sufficient for DMC purposes. However, in some cases, AE incidence may vary by geographic region due to multiregional issues discussed in Chapter 4. As one example, the control group in a clinical trial might be standard of care but the standard varies by geographic region. The statistical method off *logistic regression analysis* (Hosmer and Lemeshow 2000) can be helpful in this case. This method allows for assessing the effect of covariates on incidence. In our example, standard of care and treatment might be included as covariates in a logistic regression model. A statistical test of significance can be made to see if standard of care has an effect on AE incidence over and above treatment. If the effect is statistically significant, standard-of-care-adjusted rates can be computed and compared between treatments.

5.2.5 Laboratory Data

DMCs are often provided with listings of laboratory data—serum chemistry and urine analysis. The specific use of these data by DMCs depends on the disease and intervention. The clinical laboratory data may be of use to find the effects of treatment on analytes that may be related to renal function, heart function, anemia, and so on. The sponsor should establish laboratory ranges of normal and clinically significant changes for each blood and urine analyte at the commencement of the trial. These parameters may differ by patient age, by gender, and among laboratories if more than a single central laboratory is used. Changes in analytes from baseline or from visit to visit that are deemed clinically significant should be reported as either AEs or SAEs. Reference to a patient-by-patient listing of laboratory values and changes from baseline by DMC members will show if investigators are complying with this requirement and may turn up safety signals that are not apparent from AE and SAE reports. As the trial progresses, the DMC may wish to concentrate on particular analytes of interest and ask the DAC for listings and graphs that illustrate the dynamics of these measures over time.

5.3 Analysis Methods: Frequentist

5.3.1 What Is *Frequentist* Analysis?

Frequentist analysis is the statistical methodology that is commonly taught in statistics courses, described in textbooks, and used extensively. This application of statistics depends on repeated sampling for its measure of uncertainty and inferential basis. We will illustrate how repeated sampling plays into the frequentist statistical methods we use as we introduce each concept. We use the term "frequentist" here to distinguish these well-known methods from likelihood and Bayesian methods which do not depend on repeated sampling for inference. We will discuss these methods later in this chapter.

5.3.2 Hypothesis Tests

DMCs will often be presented *p-values* for hypothesis tests on AE incidence. The p-value is also known as the *attained significance level*. In statistical terms, the null hypothesis always states the negative result so that the null hypothesis for comparing AE incidence between two groups would usually be that there is no difference in AE frequency between experimental treatment and control in the target patient population. The alternate hypothesis might say that the frequencies are unequal—meaning either that experimental has higher frequency than control or vice versa. This is known as a *two-sided* alternative. There are two possible *one-sided* alternatives. The first would be that AE frequency in the experimental treatment is greater than that for the control treatment. The second one-sided alternative would be the opposite of this. In safety monitoring of clinical trials, DMCs would normally be interested in the former—experimental greater than control. However, under some circumstances, a two-sided alternative might be preferred. The p-value is the probability of a *Type I* error, that is, that we reject the null hypotheses (i.e., declare a treatment difference) when the null hypothesis is, in fact, true (i.e., in truth there is not a treatment difference). In designing clinical trials on the basis of efficacy endpoints, we usually set our error rate to be no greater than 0.05. This Type I error setting is called the *significance level* of the test and is usually denoted by the Greek letter alpha, α.

For the rofecoxib thrombolic event incidence data in Table 5.2, one method for computing the p-value for the difference in incidence (rofecoxib 3.57%, placebo 2.00%) is the *chi square test*. The details of computing the chi square test are contained in most statistical textbooks (see, e.g., Rosner 2006). The p-value computed for the incidence data by chi square is $p = 0.008$. This means that the probability that this difference could have arisen by chance if, in fact, incidence between rofecoxib and placebo were equal is 0.008. Another method of calculating the p-value is by Fisher's exact test (Rosner 2006). This test is implemented in many statistical software packages (see, e.g., Cytel 2007; SAS Institute 2008). For the data at hand, the one-sided p-value calculated by this method is 0.01 while the two-sided p-value is 0.015. A standard criterion for defining statistical significance is p-value less than 0.05 (known as the *significance level*). Both of our methods yield p-values of less than 0.05. Hence, we conclude that the difference in thrombotic AE incidence is statistically significant. This does not mean that the difference is clinically significant. It merely means that the difference that we have observed was not likely to have occurred due to chance. Some clinicians, acknowledging that the difference was unlikely to have occurred by chance, might feel that an incidence difference of 1.57 is not clinically meaningful. Indeed, clinicians might see a difference in incidence that they deem clinically meaningful that is not statistically significant. We will deal with that situation later in this chapter. For now, it is sufficient to remember that if the p-value were calculated to be greater than 0.05, we cannot conclude that thrombotic event incidence is equal between treatments. We can only say that we have seen no evidence of a statistically significant difference. A larger sample size might have found the observed difference statistically significant. The results of these statistical hypothesis tests are found in Table 5.3.

It is possible to test the null hypothesis of no difference between Kaplan–Meier time-to-event curves against the alternative of a difference between curves. The p-values for this hypothesis test are generated using the *log rank test* (Cox 1972; Cleves, Gould, Guttierrez et al. 2008; SAS Institute 2008). Table 5.3 indicates that the log rank test for our example has yielded a p-value of 0.008 for the treatment difference in time to first occurrence of thrombotic AE. The log rank test requires assumptions that might not be met for adverse event data. While this test might often be associated with a primary efficacy endpoint such as time to death, time to disease progression, and so on, these assumptions might not be met in safety data. The log rank test should not be the primary hypothesis test for safety data. It should be considered supportive and generated only for those AE types being followed as possible concerns.

TABLE 5.3

Statistical Inference of Adjudicated Thrombotic Adverse Event Data from the APPROVe Trial

	Rofecoxib	Placebo
Incidence (%)	3.57 (46/1287)	2.00 (26/1299)
p-Value: chi square	Chi sq = 5.907, 1 df, p = 0.008	
Fisher's exact test (one sided)	p = 0.010	
Fisher's exact test (two sided)	p = 0.015	
Log rank test	P = 0.008	
95% Confidence interval for incidence (normal approximation)	(2.56, 4.58)	(1.24, 2.76)
95% Confidence interval for incidence (exact binomial, Clopper–Pearson)	(2.63, 4.74)	(1.31, 2.92)
Incidence rate/100 patient years	1.50	0.78
95% Confidence interval for rate/100 patient years (normal approximation)	(1.07, 1.93)	(0.48, 1.08)
95% Confidence interval for rate/100 patient years (binomial approximation)	(1.11, 1.99)	(0.51, 1.14)
Relative risk and 95% confidence interval	1.76 (1.09, 2.83)	
Odds ratio and 95% confidence interval	1.82 (1.12, 2.95)	
Poisson rate ratio and 95% confidence interval (normal approximation)	1.92 (1.19, 3.11)	
Poisson rate ratio and 95% confidence interval (binomial approximation)	1.92 (1.16, 3.25)	

5.3.3 Confidence Intervals

Confidence intervals (CI) enable us to estimate a plausible range for an unknown parameter. There is a need to compute confidence intervals for our parameter estimates because we must account for the variability of estimates taken from limited samples. The degree of uncertainty decreases with increasing sample size. We now look at various methods of estimating confidence intervals for different parameters encountered in safety analysis. We will introduce some new analytic methods in the process.

5.3.3.1 Incidence

We first look at confidence intervals for the incidence estimates. There are two methods of estimating confidence intervals that we can use—the normal approximation (Rosner 2006) and exact binomial method also known as Clopper–Pearson (Clopper and Pearson 1934; Hollander and Wolfe 1999). The normal approximation works well when the number of events is greater than 15. For this reason, many DMCs prefer the exact binomial method. Table 5.3 shows that rofecoxib thrombotic AE incidence was 3.57%. The 95% confidence interval using the normal approximation, written as (lower limit, upper limit), is (2.56%, 4.58%). The interpretation of this interval is that if we were to perform this clinical trial an infinite number of times and estimated incidence and the confidence interval at the end of each trial as we have then 95% of intervals so calculated would contain the true incidence. Thus we have "95% confidence" in this interval. It is important to note that the frequentist confidence interval definition does not imply that the probability is 95% and that the true value of the parameter lies between 2.56% and 4.58%. In fact there is nothing magic about these two numbers. They are just estimates that came from one realization of a clinical trial that will be performed only once but, for probability theory purposes, we assume that it could be repeated infinitely many times. DMCs concerned about the rate of thrombotic AEs would see that a rate as high as 4.58% is within the plausible range implied by the data.

The details of computing the exact binomial confidence limit are not presented here but are presented in the references cited above. The calculations can be made with readily available software (Cytel 2007; SAS Institute 2008). The exact binomial 95% confidence interval for rofecoxib is (2.63%, 4.74%) which is pretty close to the normal approximation because the number of events was sufficiently large. Still, the binomial interval is asymmetric about the point estimate of incidence while the normal approximation interval is necessarily symmetric. Some statisticians like the elegance of the asymmetric interval. For placebo, the corresponding 95% confidence intervals are (1.24%, 2.76%) and (1.31%, 2.92%), respectively. Thus, for placebo, we have a high level of confidence that the thrombotic AE rate is less than 3.00%. This is further evidence of the separation of distributions of rofecoxib and placebo. It is consistent with the statistically significant difference we found earlier.

5.3.3.2 Rate per 100 Patient Years

If incidence is constant over time, the rate per 100 patient years follows the Poisson distribution (Rosner 2006). There are two methods for computing approximate 95% confidence intervals for the rate per 100 patient years—normal and binomial. For the normal distribution method, the standard error of the rate per 100 patient years is calculated

$$S = \frac{\sqrt{X}}{T} \tag{5.1}$$

where X = no. of events, T = patient years. If R = rate/100 patient years then the 95% CI is

$$(R - 1.96 * S, R + 1.96 * S) \tag{5.2}$$

In our example for rofecoxib, $R = 1.50$, $X = 46$, and $T = 3059$. Hence, $S = 0.22$ and the 95% CI for rate/100 patient years is (1.07, 1.93).

The binomial method consists of taking the endpoints of the exact binomial confidence limits for incidence and multiplying them by N/T where N is the sample size. For rofecoxib $N/T = 1287/3059 = 0.42$. Hence, the binomial approximation for the confidence interval for rate/100 patient years for rofecoxib would be 0.42×2.63 and 0.42×4.74 or (1.11, 1.99). For placebo, the multiplier is 0.39 (1299/3327) and the resulting 95% confidence interval is (0.51, 1.14).

Similarly for placebo, the 95% confidence interval would be (0.48, 1.08). These confidence intervals show the separation of rates between treatment groups. Our study of confidence intervals leads us to methods of estimating the relative intensity of adverse events between treatment groups: relative risk (RR), odds ratio, and the Poisson rate ratio.

5.3.3.3 Relative Risk

The *relative risk* between treatment groups is merely the ratio of incidence in the experimental group to incidence in the control group. This method is intuitive and straightforward. It is preferred by clinicians and is the recommended comparison method for prospective studies (Altman 1991; Gibbons and Amatya 2016). Relative risk is calculated as

$$RR = \frac{P1}{P2}$$

where
    $P1$ = proportional incidence in the experimental group
    $P2$ = proportional incidence in the control group

Relative risk equal to 1 indicates no association between treatment and risk of AE.

The confidence interval for relative risk can be calculated online using MedCalc (2016a). The calculations in Table 5.3 show that in our rofecoxib example, relative risk (RR) is calculated as 1.76 with a 95% confidence interval of (1.09, 2.83). Since the interval does not include unity, we can conclude that there is a statistically significant difference in incidence of thrombotic events between treatment groups with the events occurring more frequently in the rofecoxib group.

In preparing for a DMC meeting, members might glance down the list of relative risks for adverse events and flag a relative risk greater than 5, say, for further investigation. For moderate or worse adverse events, perhaps, a cutoff of 3 would flag further discussion.

Owing to the similarity of relative risk and odds ratio, much of the following discussion of odds ratio interpretation also applies to the relative risk.

A useful method of displaying relative risks graphically is presented in Section 5.8.

5.3.3.4 Odds Ratio

The *odds ratio* is a useful measure of association. In our case, it would measure the degree of association of thrombotic AEs with a treatment group. The odds ratio is recommended for use in case-control studies rather than clinical trials (Deeks 1998) but in most cases, the results are similar to those of relative risk and biostatisticians often prefer odds ratio to relative risk because the odds ratio is used in conjunction with logistic regression analysis which is described below.

The odds ratio is calculated as

$$C = \frac{P1(1-P2)}{P2(1-P1)} \tag{5.3}$$

where
$P1$ = proportional incidence in the experimental group
$P2$ = proportional incidence in the control group

An odds ratio of C equal to 1 would indicate no association (i.e., null hypothesis of no difference in AE incidence between treatments). The greater the odds ratio is greater than unity the more AE is associated with rofecoxib. An odds ratio less than 1 would indicate that the AE occurs more frequently with placebo. We see in Table 5.3 that the odds ratio in our example is calculated as 1.82 and the 95% confidence interval is (1.12, 2.95). This interval, which does not include 1, is another way of indicating that the null hypothesis is rejected in favor of greater AE incidence in rofecoxib. There are several methods for computing confidence intervals for the odds ratio and validated software is available (Gart 1970, 1971; Agresti 1992; Cytel 2007; SAS Institute 2008; Gibbons and Amatya 2016). MedCalc provides a free online calculator for the odds ratio and its confidence interval (MedCalc 2016b).

When AE tables are produced for DMC review, it is common for members to glance down the AE list looking for large odds ratios, say greater than 5. Different DMC members will have different cutoff numbers and the cutoff will depend on the nature of the disease. The purpose is to find treatment differences of interest for further discussion and follow-up. Large odds ratios that are not statistically significant are still worth noting because this may be an early signal. Some DMC members may prefer a combination of odds ratio cutoff and significance level—such as $p \leq 0.10$ and odds ratio greater than 3. Many AEs associated with large odds ratios will not be of clinical concern. The confidence intervals will shrink with increasing sample size as the trial progresses. The odds ratio may shift downward in time but trends are worth watching if the AEs are clinically important. When trends are spotted in this manner, the closed meeting minutes should note them so that members will remember to follow-up at future meetings. When the DMC is masked to treatment and receives tables classified only by coded treatment groups the control group will be unknown. In these cases, a convention can be established such that the odds ratio is always computed with Treatment A as the denominator treatment. In these cases, DMC members inspecting tables might look for either odds ratios greater than 5 or less than 0.20 in an initial screening.

Appendix Table A.1 presents adverse events observed for selected marketed drugs in placebo-controlled trials. Exact binomial 95% confidence intervals are calculated for drug and placebo incidence. The odds ratio is presented along with its 95% confidence interval. In going over the odds ratios on this list, we can get an idea of how some DMCs might have reacted to safety listings at data review meetings. For seasonal allergic rhinitis drug fexofenadine, a DMC might be concerned with the odds ratio of 5 for both dysmenorrhea and drowsiness and would also have to consider that these AEs occur at only 1.5% incidence on fexofenadine and the upper limit of the 95% confidence interval is only 2.7%. Conversely, the odds ratio of 11.3 for the adverse event of flushing for erectile dysfunction drug sildenafil might be of greater concern because sildenafil incidence is 10% reaching a 95% upper limit of 12.3%. The various adverse events listed for fibromyalgia drug pregabalin would, presumably, have generated much discussion for a DMC. Odds ratios for the selected AEs range from 4.9 to 13.6. The odds ratio of 8.3 for dizziness was associated with a 45.0% incidence in the pregabalin group with an upper limit of the 95% confidence interval of 49.1%.

5.3.3.5 Poisson Rate Ratio

Relative risk and the odds ratio are useful in inspecting AE tables to spot AE types for further discussion. Once an AE of concern emerges, DMCs should give serious consideration to computing the Poisson rate ratio.

The Poisson rate ratio is the ratio of events/100 patient years in the two groups. In the thrombotic AE example (Table 5.3), the rate ratio = 1.92 (1.50/0.78). This means that the risk per unit time is 1.92 greater for a rofecoxib patient than a placebo patient. There are two methods for computing 95% confidence intervals for the rate ratio—normal approximation and binomial approximation.

Methods for the normal approximation were derived by Ng and Tang (2005). We will be using the method they refer to as W3.

$$R = \frac{X_1/t_1}{X_o/t_o} \qquad (5.4)$$

$$Q = \ln(R)$$

$$SE(Q) = \sqrt{\left(\frac{1}{X_o}\right) + \left(\frac{1}{X_1}\right)}$$

where
  R = Poisson rate ratio
  ln = natural log function
  Q = natural log of R
  SE = standard error of Q
  X_1 = number of events in the experimental group or 0.5 if zero events
  X_o = number of events in the control group or 0.5 if zero events
  t_1 = patient years in the experimental group
  t_o = patient years in the control group

$$\text{now compute } U1 = Q - 1.96 \times SE(Q)$$
$$U2 = Q + 1.96 \times SE(Q)$$

$$\text{The 95\% CI for } R = (\exp(U1), \exp(U2)) \qquad (5.5)$$

where exp is the exponential function.

The resulting 95% confidence interval for the rate ratio of 1.92 is (1.19, 3.11).

The binomial approximation to the CI for the Poisson rate ratio conditions on the total number of events in each group, that is, assumes that we fixed this number in advance. It creates the proportion

$$P = \frac{X_1}{(X_1 + X_o)}$$

where X_1 = number of events in the rofecoxib group and X_o = number of events in the control group. Hence, in our case, P represents the proportion of thrombotic AEs that occurred in the rofecoxib group which is equal to 0.639 (46/73). This proportion has an exact binomial confidence interval of ($P1, P2$) or (0.517, 0.749). The 95% CI for the Poisson rate ratio estimated by this method is equal to ($F1, F2$) where

$$F1 = \frac{P1(d)}{1 - P1}$$

$$F2 = \frac{P2(d)}{1 - P2}$$

where $d = t_o/t_1$ with t_o and t_1 defined as above. In our example, the 95% confidence interval is (1.16–3.25). The binomial method would be preferred when the number of events is less than 50.

Both methods of computing 95% confidence intervals for the thrombotic event rate ratio yield intervals that exclude 1, leading to the conclusion of a statistically significant difference in rate ratio between treatment groups at significance level 0.05.

In practice, DMC members should glance at the listings of these AE rate ratios in a manner similar to that described for odds ratios above. The difference between these rate ratios and the odds ratios is that the rate ratios take exposure into account. This may be important when the exposure differs between the two treatment groups.

Closely related to the Poisson rate ratio is the *hazard ratio* associated with the Kaplan–Meier time-to-event graphs (Cox 1972; Cleves, Gould, Guttierrez et al. 2008; SAS Institute 2008). This ratio indicates the relative risk per unit time of a patient in one group having an event compared to another group. As for hypothesis testing, its use requires assumptions that might not be met in practice. One of these assumptions, proportional hazards, was not met for the adjudicated thrombotic AE data in APPROVe in our example (Bresalier, Sandler, Quan et al. 2005) and, hence, the hazard ratio was not calculated. The Poisson rate ratio and its confidence interval are generally sufficient as a time-corrected relative risk measure for routine safety analysis. Owing to the correction for exposure/follow-up, the rate/100 patient years is a preferable measure of incidence and the Poisson rate ratio is the preferable method for comparing incidence between treatment groups. We will see in Chapter 6 how ignoring follow-up time can lead to inferential errors. Of course, the most sophisticated method for including exposure is the Kaplan–Meier technique.

5.3.3.6 Inference with Kaplan–Meier Landmark Estimates of Incidence

Confidence intervals can be placed on the Kaplan–Meier landmark incidence using standard errors given in the Kaplan–Meier life tables and referencing the normal distribution. Similarly, hypotheses can be tested using normal distribution theory. Common methods are presented in Kaplan and Meier (1958), Rosner (2006), SAS Institute (2008), and Cleves, Gould, Guttierrez et al. (2008). Klein, Logan, Harhoff et al. (2007) present and compare several new methods based on fewer assumptions than the traditional methods.

5.3.4 Data Analysis without Statistics

For certain DMC deliberations, the use of statistical methods might be considered overkill or even misleading. One example arises often in multiregional trials where the DMC is interested in whether or not AEs are being reported more frequently by investigators in one center, country, or region than others. Disparities may be due to underperformance or cultural/medical practice differences. Reading tables organized geographically would usually be sufficient for this purpose. The DAC could compute rate ratios or odds ratios comparing regions upon request from the DMC but since the requested analysis arises only because a large AE incidence has been observed in one region and DMC members can find another region with a low incidence, the p-value or confidence interval computed would be suspect because the values compared were selected on the basis of their large difference. In any case, regardless of statistical significance, the DMC will probably want to investigate the origins and either conclude that the differences are cultural or suggest ways of bringing all investigators to a common method of medical practice (use of diagnostics, anti-infective drugs, sterilization, etc.). Inspection of tables of the use of concomitant medications and laboratory procedures for these different regions would help in this investigation and could be accomplished without statistical analysis.

5.4 Power

It is important for DMC members to understand the concept of *power*. This concept is most often used in computing the sample size for the trial on the basis of presumed data on the primary efficacy endpoint. The power is related to *Type II* error, the probability that we accept the null hypothesis of no treatment difference when it is false, that is, when there actually is a difference but we have not seen statistical evidence of this difference because our sample size is too small to have sufficient power to detect this difference. Power is a probability computed as 1—Type II error. It is important for those reviewing safety data over time to take this concept into account. Briefly stated, power is the frequentist probability of rejecting the null hypothesis of no treatment group difference when we really want to reject this hypothesis. If a placebo group has a cardiotoxicity rate of 5% and the true corresponding rate on the experimental treatment group is 10% or more, this difference would be considered clinically significant and it would be important to detect this difference in a trial (i.e., reject the null hypothesis, compute a p-value of less than 0.05). We would like the probability or the power of detecting this magnitude difference to be high, around 0.80 at least. Because of patient-to-patient variability, the smaller the sample size (number of patients in each group), the less likely we are to detect this magnitude of difference even if it really exists. At the end of the trial, there may well be enough patients to have adequate power for this hypothesis test but DMCs are looking at safety data throughout the trial. Biostatistical members of DMCs will want to ensure that the DMC does not conclude at a regular interim data review meeting that they can dismiss cardiotoxicity as an issue for this trial because the incidences of cardiotoxicity reported were placebo 3%, experimental 8%, and the p-value was 0.23. This failure to find statistical significance in the difference could be merely due to the small sample size. This is why it is only correct to say that no evidence of a statistically significant difference has been found leaving open the possibility of a different conclusion with a larger sample size. Indeed, even if a statistical significance is found between treatment groups during the trial, the discreteness of the data often indicates that one AE more or less in one of the groups would increase the attained significance level above 0.05 and the data have not been completely vetted yet.

We return to the thrombotic adverse event data in Table 5.2. Let's assume that the observed placebo rate was the expected true rate of thrombotic events for this population. With a sample size of approximately 1290 patients in both the rofecoxib group and the placebo group, the trial would have the power to detect a rate of 3.6% in the rofecoxib group (this was the observed rate) of 0.80. However, at a data review meeting with only 600 patients in each group, the DMC would have a power of 0.80 to detect a 4.6% rate on rofecoxib and with 300 patients in each group a power of 0.80 to detect a 6.00% rate. These rates are considerably larger than the clinically significant rate of 3.6%. The sample size of 600 patients would have only a power of 0.51 to detect the clinically significant rate of 3.6% in rofecoxib and the 300- patient sample size would yield a power of only 0.32. A summary of the power analysis for rofecoxib versus placebo will be found in Table 5.4.

This analysis of precision of sample size at data review meetings is sometimes called *assay sensitivity* (D'Agostino, Massaro, and Sullivan 2003). It is important that at the beginning of each closed session, the DAC biostatistician indicates the assay sensitivity, that is, the magnitude of differences from control group incidence, which the current sample size delivers in terms of power, for different levels of control group event rates. In analysis of efficacy, a Type I error may be called *regulator's risk* because the regulators would not want the hypothesis of no treatment difference to be rejected when there is, in fact, no difference. The Type II error might be called *sponsor's risk.*

TABLE 5.4

Power Analysis of Rofecoxib versus Placebo Assuming
Thrombotic Event Rate in Placebo Group Is 2.0%

Sample Size in Each Group	Rofecoxib Rate (%)	Power to Detect Rofecoxib Rate in Previous Column
1290	3.6	0.80
600	4.6	0.80
	3.6	0.51
300	6.0	0.80
	3.6	0.32

The sponsor would not want to declare no treatment difference in efficacy when, in fact, there is evidence of experimental treatment superiority over control.

If the control group were an active control rather than placebo, power would have to be calculated on a two-sided basis because we would consider event rates less than control as well as greater than control to be of clinical significance. This can be easily calculated.

Closely related to power is the concept of *conditional power.* We will take up conditional power in Chapter 7, as part of the DMC interim analysis and decision-making responsibilities.

5.5 Multiplicity

At data review meetings, the DMC is presented with long lists of AEs for many MedDRA preferred terms within body systems. As was described above, p-values and odds ratios can be computed for each. Recall that the definition of the p-value is the probability that the observed treatment difference in AEs would have occurred due to chance if there was truly no treatment difference. In a list of 100 AEs, we would, on the average, expect 5 to be statistically significant due to chance. If chance is solely responsible for the difference, we call this result a *false positive.* DMC members who make lists of AEs with small p-values (say less than 0.10) prior to the meeting will have some false positives on this list. However, further consideration of the severity of the AE, likely relationship to the disease, and so on, will often eliminate many of these AE types from concern. Indeed, there will be AE types that are serious and unexpected that have p-values of greater than 0.10 that may become the focus of discussion at the DMC closed session. The multiplicity issue does not appear to be a major problem for DMC review of AE lists because statistical significance is not a major factor in selecting AEs for concern.

In some cases, there may be interest in reducing the list of AEs worthy of further attention based solely on the statistical significance criterion. We could lower our p-value cutoff to, say, 0.001. Then, there will be fewer false positives but we run the risk of increasing the rate of *false negatives*, that is, those AEs that we think we can ignore because they were not statistically significant by our newly selected stringent requirement (0.001) but are in fact treatment related. Mehrotra and Heyse (2004) have presented an approach to controlling multiplicity in safety analysis using the concept of the *false discovery rate* (FDR). The FDR was first described by Benjamini and Hochberg (1995) as a means of controlling multiplicity. The technique has recently been generalized by Pounds and Cheng (2006). The cells of Table 5.5 represent frequencies of treatment relatedness and declarations of statistical significance that might arise from a DMC safety review table of AEs. Of course, we could never construct such a table because we do not know the "truth" about relatedness. In the table, we see that the *familywise error rate* (FWER) is the proportion of all hypothesis tests that are true (no treatment effect) but are nevertheless rejected (declared statistically significant). This is the familiar Type I error. The philosophy of the FDR is that restricting FWER is too conservative. Instead, we should look at the FDR or the proportion of all hypotheses declared statistically significant where in fact no treatment effect existed.

Mehrotra and Heyse (2004) use a two-step FDR procedure to flag adverse events as statistically significant. They call this procedure DFDR for "*Double FDR*" a term coined in their personal communication with the late Professor John Tukey. The example given is that of 40 adverse events defined by the preferred term within the body system in a vaccine clinical trial involving 296 children within the ages of 12–18 months. The naive analysis shows four adverse event types to have p-values less than 0.05. The authors describe the details of computation of the FDR-adjusted p-values. The DFDR procedure consists of setting two error rates, α_1 and α_1. First, the authors select the minimum p-value within each body system (group leaders). FDR adjustments are made to both these minima as well as the individual p-values within each body system. AEs are selected for further investigation if both the body system minimum was less than α_1 and the individual AE within

TABLE 5.5

Definition of the False Discovery Rate (FDR)

Truth of Hypothesis	Declared Not Statistically Significant	Declared Statistically Significant	Total
AE is not treatment related	A	B	n
AE is treatment related	Y	Z	N-n
Total	N-R	R	N

Note: FWER = familywise error rate = expected value of B/N (Type I error); FDR = false discovery rate = expected value of B/R.

body systems passing the first test is less than α_2. Simulation procedures show that setting $\alpha_1 = 0.05$ and $\alpha_2 = 0.10$ yields good results (i.e., FDR of less than 0.10).

FDR adjustment of p-values within a group proceeds as follows:

> Suppose there are k AEs in a group, the p-values are arranged in ascending order and the highest p-value is unadjusted. For all other p values the jth in ascending order is replaced by the minimum of (j + 1)st or (k/j) x jth (or itself).

In the example cited by Mehrotra and Heyse (2004) of the first-level FDR adjustment, the 40 AE types are reduced to 8 candidates and the second-level adjustment reduces the field to 3 finalists. Mehrotra and Adewale (2012) have modified the Mehrotra and Heyse approach to increase power.

Classification of preferred terms to the body system is somewhat arbitrary and sometimes, the same or similar terms appear within several body systems. Figure 5.4 displays another way of stratifying AEs. There are four discrete categories defined by AE seriousness (serious or not serious) and incidence (high or low). The definition of serious is that given by regulatory agencies and described in Chapter 4. Presumably, a high–low determination could be made by the DAC before each data review meeting. Table 5.6 presents data for an example of FDR adjustment using this type of stratification. The table shows the initial p-values and progressive rounds of FDR adjustment using the method described above. We see that three of the four original AE types (two SAEs and one AE) make the FDR cut. Of course, the reduction would likely be more with larger and more realistic tables.

It is important to note that under no circumstances should the FDR adjustment of p-values associated with AEs be the sole reason to eliminate any AE type from further discussion. The safety review should be driven by clinical concerns based on the knowledge of the drug and the disease process. The

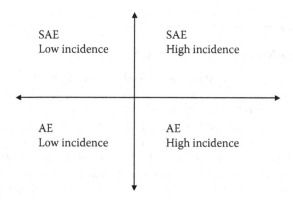

FIGURE 5.4
Stratification of adverse events by seriousness and incidence.

TABLE 5.6

Example of Use of False Discovery Rate

Group	Adverse Event Type	Initial P-Value	Group Leader FDR Adjustment ($\alpha_1 = 0.05$)	Within Group FDR Adjustment ($\alpha_2 = 0.10$)	Meets Both α_1 and α_2 Criteria
SAE high incidence	Anemia	0.02	0.03	0.06	Yes
	Renal failure	0.20		0.30	
	Anorexia	0.30		0.30	
SAE low incidence	Myocardial infarct	0.03	0.036	0.09	Yes
	Dehydration	0.12		0.18	
	Shortness of breath	0.18		0.18	
AE high incidence	Stomatitis	0.08	0.10	0.10	
	Skin rash	0.10		0.20	
	Fever	0.23		0.28	
	Nose bleed	0.28		0.28	
AE low incidence	Diarrhea	0.036	0.048	0.04	Yes
	Nausea and vomiting	0.04		0.12	
	Blurred vision	0.26		0.31	
	Bronchitis	0.31		0.47	
	Wheezing	0.40		0.50	
	Headache	0.50		0.50	

FDR adjustment is a convenient way for the biostatistician to focus discussion in the face of multiplicity.

5.6 Analysis Methods: Likelihood

Likelihood methods of analysis are based on the foundations of statistical inference but the methods have been developed for applications to biostatistical problems most recently by Royall (1997, 2000), Blume (2002), and Rohde (2014). Likelihood methodology is a useful tool of inference for DMCs because the methods yield insight on AE incidence, event rates, and relative risk conditional on the data we have observed up to the point of data review. Likelihood methods are *not* based on the repeated sampling foundation of frequentist methods. DMC use of likelihood methods will not get involved with the conundrums of multiplicity. The methods will yield a plausible range of AE incidence or event rates conditional on the data we observed not, as frequentist methods provide, based on the success rate of a formula including the true value if the clinical trial were repeated infinitely. Advocates of likelihood inference criticize frequentist methods that seek to control Type I (significance level) and Type II (related to power) errors because these errors do not measure the *evidence* gained from the clinical trial for different values of AE incidence or event rates. Only through likelihood methods can relative evidence be assessed. It is relative evidence that is central to DMC deliberations on AE incidence and event rates.

Frequentist methods are *deductive*. To take a clinical example, a deductive method would ask: given the disease what symptoms can we expect? The statistical analog to this is given the parameter of incidence, what should the data we collect look like in terms of central tendency and variation. Inference in everyday medical practice is *inductive*. Physicians are generally reasoning given the symptoms that are observed in their patient what diagnoses are most likely, moderately likely, and unlikely? Statistically given the data we have observed, what parameter values (mean AE incidence, rate/100 patient years) are most likely, moderately likely, and unlikely?

Consider the toss of a coin. We expect the probability of the coin landing head to be 0.50. This would be the definition of a "fair" coin. Suppose we toss the coin 3 times and observe three heads. We now might ask conditional on the data we observed (3 heads) what is the relative likelihood that this coin has the property of probability of head = 0.50, 0.75, and so on. This is the kind of inference we want to use for DMC data review.

Refer again to the incidence of confirmed thrombotic events in the APPROVe trial (Table 5.2). For the rofecoxib patients the event rate/100 patient years was 1.50.

The reference probability distribution for rate/100 patient years is the Poisson distribution. The likelihood function may be thought of as reflecting our relative belief in the magnitude of the parameter (mean rate) given the data collected. The log likelihood function is written as

$$\ln(\lambda \mid X, T) = -\lambda T + X \ln(\lambda) \tag{5.6}$$

where the Greek letter λ (lambda) represents the mean rate
X = total number of events
T = total patient years

From Equation 5.6, we can calculate the *maximum likelihood* (i.e., best supported by the data) value of λ, denoted as $\hat{\lambda}$

$$\hat{\lambda} = \frac{X}{T} \tag{5.7}$$

or the total number of events divided by total patient years. We multiply by 100 in order to express in rate/100 patient years. We see that the way we have been calculating this rate all along is the maximum likelihood value for this rate from the Poisson distribution.

The value of lambda for the rofecoxib arm of the APPROVe trial that has maximum likelihood is 1.50 (Table 5.2).

We now compute the log likelihood ratio for lambda. It is written as

$$A(\lambda \mid X, T) = \ln L(\lambda \mid X, T) - \ln L(\hat{\lambda} \mid X, T)$$

or Equation 5.6 with $\hat{\lambda}$ substituted in the subtraction term. The likelihood ratio for λ is then

$$LR(\lambda \mid X, T) = \exp(A(\lambda \mid X, T)) \tag{5.8}$$

(where exp denotes the exponential function), that is, the ratio of the likelihood of various values of lambda to the value of lambda with maximum likelihood. Figure 5.5 presents a graph of this ratio for various values of lambda. The graph shows the relative likelihood of a range of values of lambda. The graph reaches a maximum value of one at theta = 1.50 the maximum likelihood value. The horizontal line, drawn at 0.125 (1/8), marks the 1/8 *support level*. The line intersects the curve at 1.10 and 2.00. This range (1.10, 2.00), is called the *support interval* and is somewhat analogous to a 95% confidence interval. It represents a range of values of lambda that are reasonably supported by the data. Royall (1997) and Blume (2002) have indicated that values of theta outside of this range are weakly supported by the data collected. If DMC members have a prior concern about thrombotic events on rofecoxib, they might want to review this support interval from meeting to meeting, just to see how the data support various values of the event rate. For example,

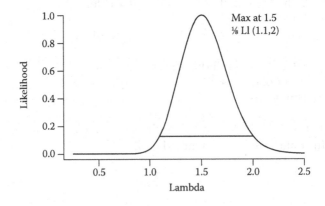

FIGURE 5.5
Likelihood support graph for rofecoxib group adjudicated thrombotic event rate per 100 patient years (lambda).

from this graph, the DMC members would conclude that, although the maximum likelihood value for rofecoxib rate is 1.50/100 patient years, the data from APPROVe support values of this rate as high as 2.00 but there is little support for values greater than 2.00. They might also want to review the support curve for the placebo group thrombotic event rate. As Figure 5.6 shows the 1/8 support interval for placebo rate is (0.51, 1.14).

We now turn to assessing evidence on relative risk or what we have been calling the Poisson rate ratio and denoting it as the Greek letter theta, θ

$$\theta = \frac{\lambda_1}{\lambda_o}$$

where
   λ_1 = event rate in rofecoxib group
   λ_o = event rate in the placebo group

In order to assess evidence of various values of theta, we must compute the relative likelihood for the ratio of rofecoxib to placebo event rates. To compute this likelihood, it is necessary to condition on the total number of events in both groups, that is, regard the total number of events as fixed, as if we specified pre-trial that there would be, in this case, a total of 72 thrombotic events at this point in the trial. Under this conditioning, the log likelihood of theta reduces to the binomial form

$$\ln L(\theta \mid X_1, X_o, T_1, T_o, N) = X_1 \ln w + (N - X_1)\ln(1 - w) \tag{5.9}$$

where
   X_1 = total events in rofecoxib group
   X_o = total events in placebo group

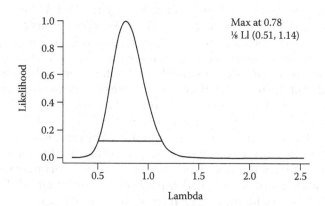

FIGURE 5.6
Likelihood support graph for placebo group adjudicated thrombotic event rate per 100 patient years (lambda).

T_1 = total patient years in rofecoxib group
T_o = total patient years in placebo group
N = total number of events = $X_1 + X_o$

$$w = \frac{\theta}{\theta + (T_o/T_1)}$$

The maximum likelihood value of theta is

$$\hat{\theta} = \frac{\hat{\lambda}_1}{\hat{\lambda}_o}$$

where $\hat{\lambda}_1$ and $\hat{\lambda}_o$ are defined using Equation 5.7 for each treatment group. The maximum likelihood value of w is

$$\hat{w} = \frac{\hat{\theta}}{\hat{\theta} + (T_o/T_1)}$$

The log likelihood ratio for theta is

$$B(\theta \mid X_1, X_o, T_1, T_o, N) = \ln L(\theta \mid X_1, X_o, T_1, T_o, N) - \ln L(\hat{\theta} \mid X_1, X_o, T_1, T_o, N)$$

and the likelihood ratio for theta is

$$LR(\theta \mid X_1, X_o, T_1, T_o, N) = \exp(B(\theta \mid X_1, X_o, T_1, T_o, N)) \qquad (5.10)$$

The likelihood graph for theta is shown in Figure 5.7. Likelihood is maximized at the observed rate ratio of 1.92. The 1/8 support limits are (1.18, 3.22). This interval indicates that conditional on the data collected to date, there is weak evidence, or support, for a rate ratio of one, the value that would represent no difference in risk. This conclusion is the same as that for frequentist methods but the interpretations are different. While the support interval reflects relative evidence conditional on the data observed, the frequentist confidence interval reflects confidence in a method of calculation because of its theoretical success rate in repeated sampling. The results of the likelihood analysis of the APPROVe trial event rates are summarized in Table 5.7.

Table 5.8 compares the confidence intervals and support intervals for the summary statistics of adjudicated thrombotic events from APPROVe. We see that there is considerable agreement in the interval across all methods of interval estimation. Royall (1997) and Blume (2002) would contend that the reason the frequentist confidence intervals have stood the test of time is because they approximate the likelihood support intervals which are

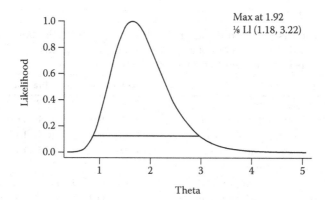

FIGURE 5.7
Likelihood support graph for the Poisson rate ratio of rofecoxib to placebo thrombotic event rates per 100 patient years (theta).

more consistent with the foundations of statistical inference than frequentist methods.

Frequentist and likelihood methods need not be an either-or. Frequentist methods can be used first. Then, for those AE treatment differences of interest, likelihood methods can be applied while discussions of correction for multiplicity are taking place. If 1/8 support intervals are to be computed for odds ratios or rate ratios for all AE types, then, DMC members may wish to concentrate on those AE types whose ratio exceeds some threshold value (say 2) and whose support intervals exclude one. Just as for frequentist methods, likelihood methods should not be the sole reason to exclude AE types from further investigation.

We have shown likelihood methods of support for the rofecoxib and placebo event rates. We could have also generated these values for the incidence rates for each treatment group and the odds ratio. The likelihood inference for incidence would use the binomial distribution as reference distribution. Royall (1997) presents several methods for computing the support intervals for the odds ratio.

TABLE 5.7

Likelihood Analysis of Thrombotic Events in the APPROVe Trial

	Rofecoxib	Placebo
Patient years	3059	3327
Number of events	46	26
Event rate/100 patient years	1.50	0.78
1/8 support limits	(1.1, 2.0)	(0.51, 1.14)
Poisson rate ratio (theta)	1.92	
1/8 support limits	(1.18, 3.22)	

TABLE 5.8

Comparison of Confidence Intervals and Likelihood Support
Intervals for Summary Statistics of Adjudicated Adverse
Events from the APPROVe Clinical Trial

	Rofecoxib	Placebo
Rate/100 patient years	1.50	0.78
95% CI—normal approximation	(1.07, 1.93)	(0.48, 1.08)
95%—binomial approximation	(1.11, 1.99)	(0.51, 1.14)
1/8 likelihood support limits	(1.10, 2.0)	(0.51, 1.14)
Poisson rate ratio (theta)	1.92	
95% CI—normal approximation	(1.19, 3.11)	
95% CI—binomial approximation	(1.16, 3.25)	
1/8 likelihood support limits	(1.18, 3.22)	

5.7 Analysis Methods: Bayesian

A complete description of Bayesian methods as applied to DMC operations in
safety review is beyond the scope of this book. The following is a description
of the difference between Bayesian methods and frequentist and likelihood
methods. Bayesian statistical methods are similar to the likelihood methods
described above but extend the inference to incorporate *prior information* on
the probability distribution of the parameter of interest such as AE incidence.
This prior information might arise from literature review, investigator brochure review, or expert opinion. If no information is available *noninforma-
tive* prior distributions can be specified (Gelman, Carlin, Stern et al. 2004).
Bayesian analysis will yield estimates of the probability that the AE incidence
is in a range or greater than some threshold value. This range estimate is
called the *credible interval* and is analogous to the frequentist confidence interval. However, the confidence interval is not conditional on the data observed
or any prior information. It is merely a success rate that the frequentist formula will have in including the parameter of interest in infinite repetitions
of the clinical trial. This estimate is based on the *posterior distribution* of the
AE inference which incorporates prior information on incidence and the data
collected in the clinical trial. Bayesian methods have been used recently in
the design and analysis of clinical trials for efficacy (Berry 2005). Berry and
Berry (2004) have applied Bayesian hierarchical methods to account for multiplicities in safety analysis. This is a Bayesian approach to the FDR methods of
Mehrotra and Heyse (2004) described above. Xia, Ma, and Carlin (2011) have
provided their own Bayesian hierarchical model approach to the analysis of
safety data. Davis and Southworth (2016) have developed a Bayesian model to
analyze annual safety update reports to create a parsimonious list of AESIs
that does not use a hierarchical listing of preferred terms.

Southworth and O'Connell (2009) compare frequentist, likelihood, Bayesian methods, and state-of-the-art data-mining methods for data-guided review of clinical trial safety data.

5.8 Safety Graphics

Graphical methods of safety data display and analysis are becoming popular. The most common graph seen by DMCs is the Amit graph (Amit, Heiberger, and Lane 2008) shown in Figure 5.8 providing a visual display of differences in incidence and relative risk and 95% confidence intervals (Gould 2013; Herson 2015a). Relative risks are presented in descending order. Volcano plots are used by some sponsors but are not yet common for DMC use (Zink, Wolfinger, and Mann 2013). Duke, Jiang, Huang et al. (2015) and Gould (2015) provide extensive galleries of graphical methods in safety and an online gallery can be found at http://www.ctspedia.org.

5.9 In Conclusion

We have described several quantitative methods for analysis of safety data. Not all of these methods will be used during the lifetime of a single DMC. The biostatistician member can work with the other DMC members and the DAC biostatistician to work out what types of data displays and statistical methods are useful for the trial at hand. Indeed, the nature of data tables and statistical methods will vary over the lifetime of the trial as safety issues come forward and are put to rest. The statistical methods guide the DMC in their deliberations but do not provide reasons to eliminate safety concerns from further discussion. A summary of statistical methods described in this chapter will be found in Table 5.9. There are many choices of statistical methods and the DMC should discuss their statistical requirements with the DAC at or shortly after the orientation meeting. Table 5.10 is a suggested list of choices of statistical methods that the DMC should discuss with the DAC prior to the start of the clinical trial. This chapter has concentrated on unmasked data analysis by the DMC. Herson (2015a) provides further analytic details for DMC data analysis but also presents the types of analyses that sponsors perform on the aggregating data with both treatment groups pooled. Our next chapter will build on our clinical and statistical knowledge to make DMC members aware of potential biases and inferential pitfalls. Chapter 7 will extend our statistical base into DMC decision making.

Data and Safety Monitoring Committees in Clinical Trials

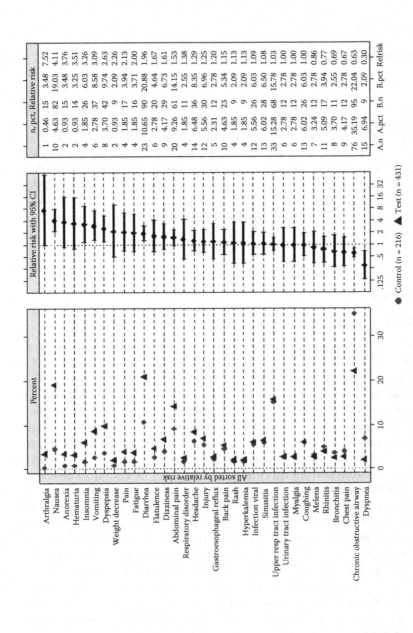

FIGURE 5.8

Amit graph of adverse event incidence by treatment and relative risk in descending order. (From Gould, A. L. 2013, personal communication; Herson, J., *Statistical Methods for Evaluating Safety in Medical Product Development*, John Wiley & Sons, Ltd., Chichester, West Sussex, 2015a.)

TABLE 5.9

Summary of Statistical Methods for Safety Analysis

Method	DMC Use	Advantages	Disadvantages
Incidence	To review the occurrence of AEs	Easy to calculate and understand	Does not take drug exposure (time on treatment) into account
Incidence rate/100 patient years	To review the occurrence of AEs per unit time	Takes both occurrence and drug exposure into account	Denominator confusing to some, does not relate to the time on treatment of any particular patient
Kaplan–Meier time-to-event graph	To graphically review the occurrence of AEs over time since treatment start	Can identify early and late risks, software readily available	Due to limitations of space not practical to be produced for every AE type
Kaplan–Meier estimate of incidence at a time point posttreatment start	To review the occurrence of AEs within a time period. One time point on a Kaplan–Meier graph	To identify patient risk within a period of time	Tendency for some people to create a crude rate by using an inappropriate denominator
p-Value	To assess probability that treatment differences in incidence could have occurred by chance if the two treatments in fact had the same incidence rates	All DMC members are familiar with the concept, software readily available	Often confused with clinical significance
Fisher's exact test, chi square test	To compute p-value for the treatment difference in incidence	All DMC members are familiar with the concept, software readily available	Chi square test not appropriate for small sample size
Log rank test	To compute p-value for the treatment difference in the Kaplan–Meier time-to-event graph	Allows for statistical assessment of the difference between curves, software readily available	Assumption of noninformative censoring often not met for safety data. Optimal only if proportional hazards assumption is satisfied
Confidence interval	To compute a range of plausible values for a parameter such as AE incidence	Allows DMC members to take sampling variation into account while assessing an AE parameter and to see if a value of interest is within the plausible range	Precise definition often not understood. Many think the interval represents the probability of the parameter lying in the interval

(Continued)

TABLE 5.9 (Continued)

Summary of Statistical Methods for Safety Analysis

Method	Purpose		
Relative risk	To assess the relative AE incidence between treatment groups	Allows for comparison of risks between treatments. Intuitive, software of confidence interval readily available	Arbitrary imputation needed when no events are observed in at least one treatment group
Odds ratio	To assess the association of AE risk and treatment group	Allows for comparison of risks, software readily available for odds ratio computation and confidence interval. Related to logistic regression	Computation not intuitive, many would prefer to compute relative risk, and arbitrary imputation needed when no events occurred in at least one group
Poisson rate ratio	To assess the relative risk of AE incidence between two treatments taking drug exposure into account	Allows for comparison of risks per unit time	Many different ways to compute the confidence interval for the rate ratio, software not readily available
Power	To assess assay sensitivity, to see how likely the sample size is to detect differences between treatments	Allows for consideration of why a statistically significant difference between treatments has not been observed	Usually separate software from that used for p-value calculation is needed. Not practical to compute for all treatment comparisons
Conditional power	To assess the power for detecting a treatment difference at a future point in time	Allows DMC to consider if a treatment difference is likely to be statistically significant at a future data review meeting	Difficult for many to understand, makes many assumptions, and software not readily available
False discovery rate (FDR)	To adjust p-values for multiplicity	Can reduce the number of AEs to consider if p-value were the chief method of prioritizing AE types for discussion	Not easily understood, may overemphasize the role of p-values in safety review, stratification methods may be seen as arbitrary, and software not readily available
Likelihood or support interval	To compute a range of plausible values of the parameter of interest conditional on the data observed	Avoids the repeated sampling interpretation of the confidence interval	Not easily understood, software not readily available
Bayesian credible interval	To compute the probability of the parameter of interest falling inside a range conditional on the data observed and on prior information	Avoids the repeated sampling interpretation of the confidence interval and incorporates prior information from previous trials or expert opinion	Not easily understood, software not readily available

TABLE 5.10

Statistical Methods to Discuss with the DAC Prior to the Start of the Clinical Trial

1. Patient years of follow-up by treatment group
2. AE incidence rate, rate/100 patient years, or both
3. Kaplan–Meier time-to-event graph for selected AE types
4. Kaplan–Meier landmark estimate for all AE types, selected AE types
5. Chi square test or Fisher's exact test
6. Include the log rank test with Kaplan–Meier graphs
7. Relative risk, odds ratio, Poisson rate ratio, or all three
8. Confidence intervals—for with point estimates and how to be computed
9. Power/assay sensitivity analysis for selected levels of AE incidence (as in Table 5.4)
10. Should DAC be prepared to calculate
    a. Simulation of projected enrollment over time
    b. Conditional power analysis
    c. False discovery rate
    d. Likelihood or support intervals
    e. Bayesian credible intervals

TABLE 5.11

Statistical Issues in the Data Review Plan

1. Shell tables, listings, and graphs to be provided, updated as trial progresses
2. Statistical methods for comparing adverse event frequency or laboratory values between treatment groups
   a. Hypothesis testing
   b. Confidence intervals
3. Criteria for extreme laboratory values requiring AE designation
4. Correction for multiplicity and/or assay sensitivity calculations in making safety comparisons
5. Extent of the use of likelihood and/or Bayesian methods

Note: See Appendix Table A.2 for a complete list of items for inclusion in the DRP.

TABLE 5.12

Potential DMC Responsibilities from This Chapter

Approve formats of tables, listings, and graphs, and statistical methods in the DRP, revise as needed

Comment on enrollment progress

Comment on safety issues in the tables, listings, and graphs

Monitor the extreme laboratory values and make sure they are also coded as adverse events when needed

Note: See Appendix Table A.3 for a complete list of DMC responsibilities.

Table 5.11 presents a list of useful items for inclusion in the DRP arising in this chapter. Table 5.12 presents a list of potential DMC responsibilities from this chapter.

Appendix Tables A.2 and A.3 display complete lists of DRP items and DMC responsibilities, respectively.

DMCounselor

Q5.1 I am a DMC Chair. Our members have been concerned that the sponsor is sending us voluminous tables to review. There are so many pages that present AEs in different ways and with maximum granularity with preferred terms. We are concerned that this information overload might mask true safety concerns.

A Your DMC has come up with an important issue. The sponsor must understand that it is the DMC that decides on the formats of reports. When huge amounts of data are issued to the DMC, it is usually because the sponsor is just dumping the same tables to the DMC that it will later submit for regulatory approval. The sponsor must be prepared to generate separate table formats for the DMC. While we are on this topic, it is useful to note that some regulatory agencies mandate that submissions for licensure break down all efficacy and safety tables by age, gender, and race. The DMC should decide at the beginning of the trials with wide eligibility requirements if they find it useful to receive tables stratified in this way.

Q5.2 I am a physician and Chair of a DMC. I have inspected the Kaplan–Meier time-to-event curves for a neurological adverse event of concern. The curves cross at the end so I have concluded that there is no difference. Our biostatistician member ignores my dismissal of this as an important event. She keeps talking about early differences. Can you explain what she is talking about?

A The important phrase of your question is "at the end." The curves will often cross at late times because there are very few patients being followed that far and the estimates are less precise than those earlier in time. Your biostatistical member is probably directing the DMC to a landmark analysis (say, 6-month posttreatment start) where she sees some evidence of a difference. This may be an event that occurs early if it is going to occur at all. She is trying to motivate discussion of this. Concentrate on estimates where the data give precise estimates as your biostatistician is correctly saying and don't worry about the tails.

Q5.3 I am the biostatistical member of a DMC working on a trial for an Infant Pharma sponsor. We have been appalled by the extremely poor quality of the data that we are receiving. The sponsor's CRO is performing poorly in monitoring, patient narratives are not arriving in a timely manner, AE forms are incomplete, and we are even concerned that the treatment group assignments may not be correct. DMC morale is low. Can we all just resign from this mess?

A The situation is clearly not acceptable but you must hesitate to resign. The DMC is responsible for the stewardship of the trial. You are there to protect patient safety and you must consider how this important function will be fulfilled if you were all to exit. The DMC must bluntly describe its expectations for data quality and indicate that your expectations are no lower than those of the regulatory agencies who will ultimately review the data. You may want to provide deadlines for improvement of certain processes and you may want to go as far as recommending that a new CRO be retained. If there is no improvement, then the DMC should recommend trial termination.

Q5.4 I am the biostatistical member of a DMC. At our organizational meeting, I requested that odds ratios and their confidence interval be computed for all treatment comparisons in safety. We just completed our second data review meeting and the DAC is merely providing p-values for the treatment difference despite my repeated requests. The physician members of the DMC show no interest in this matter. Should I just be satisfied with what I am getting or should I continue to press for what I think would be of help to me and the DMC?

A Once again, the DAC does not specify the data presentation or analysis for a DMC. This is the DMC's responsibility. As the biostatistical member, it is your responsibility to see that the analysis is done the way you think best and your fellow DMC members should support you on this just as you would support a physician member who has requested a more detailed analysis of QTc interval. You and the Chair of your DMC should approach the sponsor and tell them that you are expecting the odds ratios to appear in the tables. The sponsor should investigate what the problem is in meeting your request and get back to you with a plan for resolution. This problem can likely be avoided by an agreement at the beginning of the trial that the DMC must approve all report templates before DAC programming can commence. Also, as a biostatistical member, you should ask to see draft tables about three weeks before each meeting to make sure that they meet the requirements. There should be no surprises regarding table layout at the time of the meeting.

Q5.5 I am the DAC biostatistician on a cervical cancer clinical trial where overall survival is the principal efficacy endpoint. At the last DMC meeting I attended, it was noted that the new institutions just brought into the trial are having a lot of early deaths but they are occurring equally in both treatment groups. The biostatistical member didn't say anything. He seems to be satisfied on a safety basis because deaths are equal in both groups but I know that with a lot of early deaths in both groups, the sponsor is losing power for the ultimate hypothesis test on overall survival. I mentioned this to the statistical member after the meeting but he just said that the interim analysis of survival is still 6 months away. He may not understand what I am talking about. I am not sure that I was supposed to comment in the first place but am unsure that to do now.

A   I think you were right to talk to the biostatistical member separately and am sorry that your first attempt to bring this to his attention drew that response. If the sponsor is viewing only pooled data, they have no idea that the early deaths are occurring equally in each group so you must be careful not to unmask the sponsor. Given that this is an oncology trial they are probably unmasked anyway. Either you or the DMC Chair can certainly tell the sponsor that you are concerned about the performance of the new institutions because of the early deaths. These institutions may be admitting patients that are somehow ineligible but will, nevertheless, be included in the intent-to-treat analysis and the last thing they need to do is lose power. Even worse, the new centers may be giving inadequate care. The biostatisical member should have the first crack at articulating the power problem. I would suggest you call this person and go over the problem statistician to statistician. I am sure that he will understand and bring up the power issue while the sponsor is evaluating investigator performance at these new institutions.

Q5.6   I am the biostatistical member of a DMC working on a confirmatory trial in lymphoma. I received the package of tables, listings, and graphs for our teleconference DMC meeting 8 days before the meeting. Four days before the meeting, I had a question for our DAC biostatistician, which I asked by sending him an e-mail. I received an automated reply that he was on vacation and would not return until the day of our meeting. Nobody else at the DAC could be unmasked so there was no one else to answer my question. Shouldn't the DAC biostatistician always be available during the countdown to the meeting?

A   Of course you are right. The supervisor of the DAC biostatistician should not have allowed him to go on vacation on the days leading up to the meeting. This is especially true since DMC members will be reading the preparatory material at precisely that time. This may seem elementary but the best way to prevent this is by making sure it is understood that this support must be in place from the time the material is sent until the meeting is completed.

6

Bias and Pitfalls

PREVIEW We define bias as an observed treatment difference due to effects other than the treatments themselves. Certain analytic pitfalls will be introduced as well. Biased estimates of treatment differences can be induced by unmasking (de facto or deliberate), differential reporting of AEs between treatment groups, granularity in AE tables, competing risks, and incomplete follow-up. Spontaneous collection of adverse events might result in an underreporting of certain event types. Suggestions are given for minimizing bias and preventing inferential pitfalls.

KEY WORDS: *add-on design, bias, competing risks, de facto unmasking, deliberate unmasking, firewall, granularity bias, pitfalls, solicited AE collection, spontaneous AE collection*

6.1 What Is Bias?

In Chapter 1, we defined bias on an operational level. More scientifically, bias is a systematic difference between treatment groups in a clinical trial due to effects other than the treatments themselves (Pocock 1983). Piantadosi (2005) defines bias as a systematic (nonrandom) error in the estimate of a treatment difference. He goes on to further define bias as a state of mind based on opinion or perception that predisposes actions or evaluations in a nonobjective manner. It is the DMC's task to separate signal from noise. It will be important to consider bias as a carrier of noise. In this chapter, we concentrate on sources of bias that can create distorted treatment differences in safety. There are other pitfalls to interpretation of data which do not meet the precise definition of bias but will be covered in this chapter as well and the term "bias" will be used to apply to all sources of inferential pitfalls.

6.2 Sources of Bias

Sackett (1979) defined several sources of bias that can enter clinical research. In clinical trials, we are familiar with sources of bias such as selection bias, publication bias, observer bias, early termination bias, and so on. In what follows, we concentrate on those sources of bias that a DMC might come across in safety monitoring. These biases are of two types—knowledge of treatment assignment and underreporting.

6.3 Knowledge of Treatment Assignment

6.3.1 By Sponsor Staff

If sponsor staff is aware of treatment assignment, they might classify SAEs differently or take some actions that will cause bias. Under most circumstances, the sponsor staff working on the trial will be masked to treatment assignment until the end of the trial. The DAC will prepare reports for the DMC using coded treatment groups regardless of the DMC masking policy. At data review meetings, sponsor staff will see only pooled treatment group information. Pharmacovigilence staff at the sponsor will normally be unmasked to SAEs but there will be a "firewall" between them and the staff working on the trial meaning that the treatment assignments will not be revealed to trial staff. For Infant Pharma, CROs will often perform the pharmacovigilence function because all Infant Pharma staff may be involved with the trial. Back in the 1980s, sponsors were asking FDA permission to take "administrative looks" at the accumulating data. This would entail an interim look at efficacy and safety data by treatment group. Sponsors claimed that these looks were to plan future trials, plan for building manufacturing facilities, plan training of sales staff, and so on. FDA now frowns on this activity especially when performed by Infant Pharma sponsors (O'Neill 2007).

Even with masking, there are some analyses of extremes that can be performed by sponsors to weigh the potential of a statistically significant treatment difference in SAE incidence. For example, in the trial of lapatinib plus capecitabine (L + C) versus capecitabine alone (C) for patients with HER2-positive advanced breast cancer (Geyer, Forster, Lindquist et al. 2006), there were 164 patients randomized to L + C versus 152 randomized to C. Using Fisher's exact test, sponsor staff could determine that SAEs that occur with a frequency of 5/164 on L + C and 0/152 on C would yield a one-sided p-value of 0.037. However, a combination of 4/164 versus 0/152 would yield a one-sided p-value of 0.07. The latter would be consistent with a pooled treatment incidence of 4/316 or 1.3%. Thus, if sponsors see SAEs with pooled treatment incidence of 1.3% or greater and are confident that these SAEs are rarely or never associated with treatment by capecitabine alone, they would know that there is a chance of a statistically significant higher incidence in the combination treatment. For pooled incidence of 1.3% or less, a statistically significant difference between treatment groups would be impossible. For this trial, the authors report a pooled incidence of 5/316 or 1.6% for both asymptomatic cardiac events and fatal AEs. After doing the calculation described above, the sponsor might ask the DMC at a data review meeting if there is a concern about SAEs of these types. It is not clear how much bias this process introduces.

If sponsor staff are unmasked, their subconscience can cause them to be more aggressive in contacting investigators for "clarification" when the terms "related to study drug" or "unexpected" are used for the experimental drug rather than they would be if these terms were reported for a control subject. Pharmacovigilence staff members are usually unmasked and they must be careful to avoid this practice. Sponsor staff closer to the trial are usually unmasked for oncology trials and may become unmasked as they observe telltale adverse event patterns. DMC members should feel free to inquire about the possibility of these practices.

Sponsor MedDRA coding practices can also introduce bias. One source is granularity in classification which is discussed below under bias potential at the analysis level.

6.3.2 By the DMC

Some DMCs will choose to be unmasked to treatment from the start of their trial in case they are called upon to make decisions of risk versus benefit. There is also the feeling that DMCs should always be unmasked because this is necessary for their stewardship and is consistent with the trust put into them by the sponsor. In oncology and epilepsy the *add-on* design is common. In this design Treatment X, an approved drug for the indication is compared with Treatments X + Y where Y is an experimental treatment. When this design is used, knowledge of treatment assignment might help separate safety issues between X and Y.

When DMCs are masked to treatment, the treatments will be presented as merely A or B. There are two types of DMC unmasking that can take place during a trial—*de facto* and *deliberate*. By de facto, we mean treatments easily recognizable by the adverse event patterns that emerge as the trial progresses. Sometimes, treatment arms will involve different schedules or types of radiotherapy or surgery thus giving away treatment assignment. Also, if patients randomized to experimental treatment will receive infusions but those randomized to placebo will not undergo infusion or if placebo infusion will consist only of saline, then, the AE "infusion reactions" can unmask the DMC to the treatment group. In this case, infusion reactions can be presented only for all treatment groups combined. When 2:1 randomization is used or in oncology trials treatment group identity will be obvious. De facto unmasking also affects investigators and patients. Both receive lists in their investigator brochures and informed consent documents of adverse events to expect. If the control group is placebo, de facto unmasking is more likely to take place because all the adverse event warnings would likely apply to the experimental group. If the control group is active control, the lists of expected AEs would be written to include the union for the two treatments without designating which applies to which treatment. However, investigators would certainly know the differentiation and it would not take long for patients to gain the knowledge. DMC members might want to make sure that the routine AE tables include treatment comparisons for those adverse event types that would have an unmasking potential. For a trial where an active vaccine (injected) is compared to a placebo injection, DMC members might want to see tabulations of redness, induration, and pain at the injection site. If the DMC observes a large difference in incidence between experimental and control group, the members might be on guard for unmasking.

Deliberate unmasking refers to a decision by DMC members reviewing adverse events with coded treatments to ask the DAC statistician to unmask them to treatment assignment of the individual patients who experienced that adverse event. More will be said about this procedure in Chapter 7. Although a trial may begin with a DMC masked to treatment identity, the DMC may change their policy to be unmasked at any time during the trial.

In pharmaceutical industry trials, there is no evidence that DMC unmasking either de facto or deliberate has contributed any measurable amount of bias to their operations.

6.4 Reporting Bias

Reporting bias refers to the conscious or unconscious over or underreporting of adverse events. We will see various ways where this may occur. However, it is not the DMC's job to ensure precise estimates of AE incidence. The DMC is looking for signal among noise. For that goal, it is important for DMC members to be aware of reporting bias.

6.4.1 Investigator Level

6.4.1.1 Knowledge of Treatment Assignment

Clear knowledge of treatment assignment can cause investigators to report AEs with either greater or less frequency or assign relatedness or severity classifications to AEs differently then they would otherwise. They might be very wary of the experimental treatment and overreport. When the control group is an active control, they might feel that the safety profile for this drug is well understood and fail to report AEs. For the latter, DMC members should consult the package insert for the active control and compare the incidence for the particular AE with that observed in the trial. The biostatistician member might want to use the higher incidence to be conservative. Fay, Huang, and Twum-Danso (2007) have recently reported on a method to test the statistical significance of SAE incidence for a clinical trial with that of a historical control. This method might be appropriate for this application. Clearly one can posit alternative scenarios for AE reporting level based on investigator knowledge of treatment assignment. This is why many sponsors recommend masking.

6.4.1.2 Incomplete Follow-Up

When a trial ends for early termination due to efficacy, there may be incomplete follow-up on adverse events because investigators feel that the trial is over, are faced with considerable busy work to close the trial, and must now devote more time to other responsibilities. Similarly, in oncology trials when progression-free survival (PFS) is the primary efficacy endpoint and the trial progresses to the end with a statistically significant treatment effect in PFS, some have observed that further follow-up for overall survival, a secondary endpoint is sloppy (Temple 2003). This might also result in underreporting of AEs. DMC members should insist on complete follow-up and ask the sponsor to provide evidence that AE reporting and follow-up was complete.

6.4.1.3 Spontaneous versus Solicited Adverse Event Collection

Spontaneous AE collection is performed when, during clinic visits, the physician or nurse asks the patient to recall what events they may have experienced since their last visit. When AE data are collected by the *solicited* manner, the data collector goes down a checklist of potential AEs asking the patient to respond to those experienced. Some investigators may probe patients for adverse events that are expected. This is particularly true for approved active control drugs. Sponsors feel that solicitation is needed when there are long periods between clinic visits when patients may forget AEs that were transient and of short duration. Solicited methods are also advocated by sponsors when potentially embarrassing AEs, such as sexual dysfunction, are expected or when the clinical trial involves a treatment for a psychiatric indication such as dementia where memory is expected to be a problem. Wernicke, Faries, Milton et al. (2005) studied three randomized placebo-controlled trials which employed both methods and compared the results. Not surprisingly, reporting rates for AEs were higher in solicited collection than spontaneous but spontaneous methods were more effective in distinguishing experimental–placebo differences. DMC members should be aware of bias according to the type of data collection and should be aware of how which method is being used in the trial for which they have stewardship. This type of bias would not apply to SAEs that are expected to be reported due to the supportive care required.

The adverse events reported for osteoporosis drugs risedronate and teriparatide in Appendix Table A.1 are of interest. The placebo incidence of arthralgia for risedronate was 23.7%, higher than for risedronate incidence. For teriparatide the placebo arthralgia rate was 8.4%. Arthralgia might be present as part of the disease process. The difference in placebo incidence between trials might be due to different eligibility requirements between the trial but it might also be because the risedronate trial used solicited adverse events and the teriparatide used spontaneous reporting. Which method was used in each trial is unknown.

Owing to their importance, adverse events of special interest (AESI) and Tier 1 adverse events should always be collected in a solicited manner rather than depend on spontaneous reporting. DMC members might want to advise the sponsor on this issue.

6.4.2 Analysis Level

6.4.2.1 Early Termination Due to Efficacy

Early termination of a trial due to efficacy might also provide bias on the analysis level. If a trial terminates at a planned interim analysis, the DMC can now compare treatment groups for safety and find no important treatment differences. However, the failure to find differences might be because the sample size is not large enough to find a difference. The biostatistician member of the DMC can compute power and assay sensitivity as described in Chapter 5 to provide a quantitative assessment of potential bias. However, the DMC may suggest continuing to enroll patients on the experimental treatment and reaching a reasonable exposure time in order that the drug's safety profile can be best described. The number of patients in the control group will not increase but, depending on the disease and safety issues, may be sufficient for comparison. If desirable, the control group can be expanded by meta-analysis. This method will be described in Chapter 7 as will the methods of early termination at planned interim analyses.

6.4.2.2 Granularity Bias

Granularity refers to the number of MedDRA preferred terms listed in data review tables within a system organ class (SOC). Table 6.1 represents such a table from an infectious disease trial. Here, there are nine preferred terms within the SOC "eye disorders." For the SOC "cardiovascular disorders" there may be 50 preferred terms listed. This granularity is created when the DAC generates tables listing all preferred terms within an SOC that had at least one occurrence in either treatment group. There is concern that excess granularity may hide a signal.

Table 6.1 shows that there is a statistically significant difference in eye disorder incidence overall between treatments A and B by Fisher's exact test (one sided). However, there is not a statistically significant difference for any of the preferred terms. Suppose this committee retained an ophthalmologist member because of expected eye-related AEs. This person might say that

TABLE 6.1

Incidence of Adverse Events for MedDRA System Order Class Eye Disorders by Treatment Group and Preferred Term

	A (n = 440)	B (n = 440)	p-Value (One Sided) If p < 0.05 by Fisher's Exact Test
Any event within class	4	17	0.003
By preferred term:			
1. Chorioretinal disorders	1	0	
2. Conjunctival hemorrhage	1	2	
3. Conjunctival edema	0	2	
4. Conjunctivitis	1	5	
5. Eye inflammation	1	0	
6. Eye edema	0	2	
7. Eye redness	0	2	
8. Keratoconjunctivitis sicca	0	2	
9. Scleral edema	0	2	

the overall treatment difference is difficult to interpret because the preferred terms are heterogeneous. Tables 6.2 and 6.3 show two attempts at grouping the preferred terms to display adverse events by inflammation type and tissue type, respectively. Each table of these tables produces one subgrouping with a statistically significant difference.

The problem occurs when DMC members are unmasked either de facto or deliberately. There may be a subconscious attempt to hunt for subgroupings that provide a rationale for the difference when there is general agreement that the overall difference is meaningless because the preferred terms are heterogeneous. The problem is compounded when two specialists disagree on the grouping and even the same specialist might group preferred terms differently on two different occasions. This scenario can also occur when there is no evidence of a statistically significant difference for the SOC overall but specialists engage in preferred term clumping to seek statistically significant differences.

TABLE 6.2

Incidence of Adverse Events in Table 6.1 Grouped by Preferred Terms Representing Inflammation Types

Groupings Representing Inflammation Types	A (n = 440)	B (n = 440)	p-Value (One Sided) If p < 0.05 by Fisher's Exact Test
1,7	1	2	
2	1	2	
8	0	2	
3,4,5,6,9	2	11	0.011

TABLE 6.3

Incidence of Adverse Events in Table 6.1 Grouped by Preferred Terms Representing Types of Tissue Involved

Groupings Representing Types of Tissue Involved	A (n = 440)	B (n = 440)	p-Value (One Sided) If p < 0.05 by Fisher's Exact Test
1	1	0	
9	0	2	
2,3,4,8	2	11	0.011
5,6,7	1	4	

Obviously, a considerable amount of time can be spent in these discussions and this activity may cause the DMC to request that representatives of other medical specialities be retained as consultants to give input in combining preferred terms that occur in SOCs within their specialty. While the latter is rarely done, many DMC members wonder if there is some hidden signal within the noise introduced by granularity in preferred terms.

Goldman (2002) discusses the art and science of MedDRA coding especially pointing out biases that can occur in the process. He points out that the appropriateness of the terms "expected" and "unexpected" can depend on the degree of granularity in classification. This could result in an SAE being coded as an AE. He worries that the term "congestive heart failure" can be bypassed by merely coding the patient as having "dyspnea," "orthopnea," and "fatigue." If an investigator used only two of these three terms, it is more likely that congestive heart failure would not appear as a signal. The degree of sponsor aggressiveness in clarifying this issue with investigators could depend on whether or not they have knowledge of patient treatment group. Similarly, White (1998) observes that a strategy of intense "splitting" (granularity) can keep SAEs off of the label for the product postapproval.

Granularity bias can be minimized using standard MedDRA queries (SMQs) described in Chapter 4, using sponsor proprietary queries or at least if the DMC members and sponsor representatives can agree on preferred term combinations before the start of the trial based on expected AEs, mode of action, and pathways associated with the experimental drug. If there can be agreement as to which AE types would undergo statistical analysis of the sort shown in Tables 6.1 through 6.3 at the start of the trial, the biostatistical member can suggest analyses to control multiplicity problems. As the trial progresses and the safety profile is better understood, less granularity may be needed than was thought necessary at the beginning of the trial. Kubler, Vonk, Belmel et al. (2005) suggest the establishment of minimum incidence required for each level of specificity. For example, for 1% incidence, perhaps, only the system organ class (SOC) could be presented, for 5%, the preferred terms (unique medical concepts) could be displayed. This might ensure that there are enough patients for subclassification.

In the presence of a long list of subclassifications, DMC members might ask if the direction of differences trends toward a certain treatment. In Table 6.1, DMC members might ask if there is a trend in treatment differences in AE incidence in the direction of Treatment B. Of 9 subcategories, there are 7 in which Treatment B has a higher count of eye disorders than Treatment A. The biostatistician member of the DMC might want to refer to the binomial distribution with a null hypothesis that the probability of Treatment B having a higher count than Treatment A for any subcategory is 0.50. The probability of observing 7 or more differences in the direction of Treatment B out of 9 subcategories is 0.09. Thus, there is some evidence of a trend but the difference is not statistically significant at the 0.05 significance level.

There are no approaches to granularity bias that apply to all contexts but DMC should be guided by seriousness, severity, relatedness, unexpectedness, and so on, taking investigator brochure information on the mode of action, pathways, and so on, into account. This should not be thought of as strictly a statistical issue.

6.5 Competing Risks

Consider a hypothetical lung cancer clinical trial. The control group is Treatment A, an already-approved drug and the experimental group is Treatment A plus experimental drug B. The primary efficacy endpoint is progression-free survival (PFS) meaning that patients go off study if they die and/or show evidence of disease progression. Table 6.4 presents data on the frequency of cardiac SAEs from an interim analysis in such a trial.

TABLE 6.4

Cardiac Serious Adverse Events by Treatment Group, Interim Analysis Results from a Hypothetical Clinical Trial for Lung Cancer

	Treatment A n = 150 Patient Years = 175	Treatments A + B n = 150 Patient Years = 85	Analysis
No. of cardiac SAEs	8 (5.33%)	1 (0.67%)	p = 0.018, one-sided Fisher's exact test OR = 8.39, 95% CI: 1.04–67.97
Cardiac SAEs/100 patient years	4.57	1.18	RR = 3.89, 95% CI: 0.49, 31.07

The typical analysis would ignore patient years of follow-up as shown in the first line of the table. The incidence of cardiac SAEs for Treatment A was 8/150 (5.33%) and for A + B 1/150 (0.67%). The one-sided Fisher's exact test shows this difference to be statistically significant (p = 0.018). Some DMC members might conclude that this indicates that although Treatment A is associated with cardiac SAEs, Treatment B may have a protective effect on cardiotoxicity.

However, if we look at the patient years of follow-up, we see that the active control has 175 years and the experimental treatment has only 85 years. Further investigation might show that patients on the experimental treatment are exiting the trial sooner due to disease progression or death. Thus, the Treatment A + B patients are perhaps not exposed to their drug long enough to experience cardiotoxicity. This is an example of *competing risks*. Loosely defined, the competing risk phenomenon occurs when a patient can experience several types of events but the occurrence of one (in our case treatment failure) lowers the probability of observing another event (cardiac SAE).

If we include patient years of follow-up in our analysis and compute the number of events/100 patient years, Treatment A has 4.57 versus compared to 1.18 for Treatments A + B. The relative risk (RR) is 3.89 (4.57/1.18). With reference to the Poisson distribution the 95% CI is 0.49–31.07. This interval includes 1 and, thus, this difference is not statistically significant. The failure to attain statistical significance is due to the large variance component introduced by the shorter follow-up in the experimental arm. This is an example of why it is important for DMC members to review at every meeting a table of frequency of discontinuation by reason and treatment group and for the DAC to report patient years of follow-up by treatment group. In practice, this particular clinical trial might meet the conditions for early termination due to efficacy at the next planned interim analysis but competing risks should always be addressed as a source of bias in comparing treatment groups for safety.

A more precise safety comparison taking follow-up into account would be a Kaplan–Meier time-to-event analysis. However, neither the latter nor the Poisson analysis described previously correct the treatment comparison for competing risks. Gray (1988) presents a method of time-to-event analysis correcting for competing risks. A good overview of competing risk methods is presented by Pintilie (2006).

The analysis performed above was not planned and, as has been emphasized previously, the safety issues that arise are not strictly statistical matters. Despite the competing risks, there might very well be a protective effect of Treatment B on cardiotoxicity and this characteristic would have emerged had patients been followed longer on the experimental arm. Clinical knowledge is very important here. All we can conclude statistically is that there is no evidence of a statistically significant difference. This leaves open other interpretations and conclusions from other trials with longer follow-up.

6.6 In Conclusion

We have seen the various sources of bias and how they may be minimized. Other sources of bias may appear during the conduct of a clinical trial and DMC members should be considering this possibility in their deliberations.

TABLE 6.5

Summary of Recommended Actions to Reduce Bias

Source	Description	Action
Knowledge of Treatment Assignment		
Sponsor staff	Possible bias in classification of SAEs on experimental treatment	Separate pharmacovigilence unit at sponsor independent of clinical trial staff
DMC members	Bias in interpretation of safety data	Not considered a problem. DMC should be unmasked from the start of the trial
Investigator	Bias in reporting AEs	Masking preferable, if not compare reported AEs with label for active control, compare treatment groups for those AE types that have an unmasking potential
Incomplete Follow-Up		
Early term due to efficacy	Poor safety follow-up	DMC should work with sponsor to ensure complete follow-up
	Lack of power	DMC should calculate assay sensitivity in assessing a treatment difference in safety; perhaps perform meta-analysis
Spontaneous versus solicited adverse event collection	Solicitation of adverse events from checklists can create overestimates	Investigate how solicitation might affect the difference between experimental and control groups. Should have no effect on SAEs
Granularity	To many preferred terms under a system organ class makes it difficult to find treatment differences and can hide SAEs	DMC and sponsor should agree on meaningful preferred terms as start of the trial; binomial analysis of the trend; and minimum incidence requirement for subclassification
Competing risks	Patients exit one treatment early due to treatment failure and thus are not on study long enough to develop AEs	Analyze reasons for discontinuation, report patient years of follow-up for each treatment group, Poisson, or time-to-event analysis

TABLE 6.6

Useful Items for the Data Review Plan

List which AEs are collected by the solicited method. Assume that all others are spontaneous reporting
Note competing risk issues, update as observed

Note: See Appendix Table A.2 for a complete list of useful information for the Data Review Plan.

TABLE 6.7

Potential DMC Responsibilities from This Chapter

Suggest new SMQs (standard MeDRA queries) to reduce granularity for adverse events
Beware of competing risks

Note: See Appendix Table A.3 for a complete list of DMC responsibilities.

A summary of types of bias and recommended actions to minimize bias can be found in Table 6.5. Table 6.6 presents some useful items for the Data Review Plan. Table 6.7 presents some potential DMC responsibilities arising in this chapter. A complete list of DRP items and DMC responsibilities will be found in Appendix Tables A.2 and A.3, respectively.

In our next chapter, we take our knowledge of statistics, clinical issues, and bias to DMC decision making.

DMCounselor

Q6.1   I was asked to serve on a DMC for an Infant Pharma company. The medical director told us at our first meeting that he can be unmasked at any time. The venture capitalists agree with him. Should I serve on this DMC?

    A   This is not an uncommon occurrence in Infant Pharma. Both the executive staff and the investors are not accustomed to the rigors of good clinical practices but they understand the need to terminate trials early that may never approach statistical significance or where there may be a legal risk due to safety concerns. You ought to explain to them the credibility and statistical problems they will face by being unmasked and refer them to consultants who may help them draw up planned interim analyses. If they insist on being unmasked, then, you may have to turn down their offer to serve.

Q6.2   I am a biostatistical member of a DMC for an experimental treatment for acne vulgaris. We are masked to treatment assignment and have no efficacy responsibilities. Treatments are only identified as A, B. Whenever we see an odds ratio for an SAE of 1.5 or greater, one dermatologist member insists on being unmasked regardless of statistical significance. He is not comfortable in assessing risk unless he knows what A, B are. He claims other DMCs he has served on have always unmasked for SAEs.

A It appears that the member is not asking to be unmasked for just the treatments of those patients experiencing the SAEs. He is asking to know what A, B stand for. This member may be overly conservative about SAEs because of the controversy over isotretinoin and depression (Magin and Smith 2005). It is not clear why this person takes an odds ratio of 1.5 as a cutoff. In assessing risk when unmasked, DMC members would usually have to have access to efficacy information so that risk versus benefit could be assessed. If one member is uncomfortable being masked, it is probably best for the whole committee to be unmasked taking precautions to avoid bias. Given that all members will now be aware of what Treatment A, B stand for, it would also be important to ascertain what process this member will go through in assessing risk in the absence of efficacy data whenever an odds ratio exceeds 1.5 regardless of statistical significance.

Q6.3 I am serving as a biostatistical member of a DMC for a pediatric solid tumor clinical trial. Our Chair is a pediatrician and a world-renowned expert in pediatric oncology. At a recent meeting, she pointed out a treatment difference in renal adverse events and I pointed out that this observed difference could easily be a consequence of competing risks because patients in the arm with a lower level of renal events are also exiting the trial sooner due to treatment failure. Her reply was that we don't see competing risks in children and went on to other business. I took the floor again trying to explain that competing risks were not a function of the disease process but a statistical artifact. At this point, the other physician members of the panel followed our Chair and went on to other business. Should I complain to the sponsor?

A No, don't bring up closed meeting information to the sponsor. This is something that you must work out within the DMC. You could ask the Chair to explain why "we don't see competing risks in children." Her reply should indicate to all that she is confusing competing risks with some other phenomenon. In explaining the statistical issue, you should mention that you respect her knowledge of pediatric oncology but she must respect your knowledge of statistics. In some diplomatic way, you might remind her that statistics is your responsibility. Both clinical and statistical expertise must be represented on this committee. Come prepared with examples of competing risks, perhaps from published clinical trials in pediatric oncology, to illustrate your point. It is not likely that this problem will persist.

Q6.4 I chair a DMC for a prostate cancer clinical trial. I receive the minutes of the Steering Committee (SC) for this trial and I see the Chair of this committee put in the minutes that the committee is pleased that there is very little toxicity seen in the pooled treatments for the age 75+ group. Our DMC discussed this in closed session and thought that the SC had ignored the effect of the screening phase for this trial. About 30% of patients fail the screening phase. It is possible that only the healthiest 75+ gentlemen passed screening and those vulnerable to toxicity were screened out. We called this to the attention of the sponsor representative who replied only that the screening program is very efficient and state of the art. He obviously missed the point. Should we bother to pursue this? We didn't think it was our job to educate the SC and sponsor on bias and pitfalls.

A You and your DMC are correct about the potential bias of the screening phase. The sponsor may have given you that reply because they don't want to investigate the profile of the 75+ patients who were screened out or that such an investigation is likely to be inconclusive. It probably makes no sense for the DMC to take this on as a mission. The good news is that if this drug is approved the older postmarket patients might have the same characteristics as those screened of your trial. Hence, we might very well see little toxicity postmarket in this oldest age group. This might have been what the Chair of the SC had in mind but I wouldn't blame you if you don't give him the benefit of the doubt.

7

Data Monitoring Committee Decisions

PREVIEW This chapter describes the environment and methods surrounding actual DMC decisions. It must be kept in mind that all DMC decisions are advisory to the sponsor. DMC safety decisions are made without knowledge of efficacy. In voicing safety concerns, the DMC must be careful not to unmask the sponsor. We will describe planned interim analysis methodology used for early termination of trials for efficacy or futility as well as a "quick and dirty" method for risk versus benefit assessment. In presenting the pros and cons of bringing outside data into DMC decisions, we introduce the method of meta-analysis which is increasingly used to summarize efficacy and safety data across clinical trials.

KEY WORDS: *alpha-spending function, binding futility analysis, conditional power, "Dear Investigator" letter, futility, Haybittle–Peto, Lan–DeMets, meta-analysis, NNH (number needed to harm), NNH/NNT ratio, NNT (number needed to treat), nonbinding futility analysis, O'Brien–Fleming, planned interim analysis, PRISMA statement, publication bias, risk versus benefit*

7.1 Types of DMC Decisions

We have now learned about the DMC's role in a confirmatory trial safety monitoring program, clinical issues, statistical issues, and sources of bias. We now turn to how these issues interact when the DMC has to make decisions. The DMC decision most on the mind of sponsors and DMC members is the recommendation to terminate a trial due to safety or persuasive evidence of efficacy or *futility* (i.e., it is very unlikely that, if continued, this trial would conclude with evidence of efficacy). Termination for efficacy or futility is based on *planned interim analyses* using sophisticated statistical methods. We will describe the DMC's role in this type of decision later in this chapter. Other decisions involve the need to write a *"Dear Investigator" letter* informing investigators of potential risk, and recommending changes in the informed consent document. At the end of the trial, the DMC might be asked to review the integrated summary of safety in the regulatory submission, manuscripts presenting results of the trial, and the proposed drug label or package insert.

A quorum is usually sufficient to hold a DMC meeting but most DMC members agree that before any decision can be considered finalized all members must be consulted.

It is important to note that all DMC decisions are *advisory*. The sponsor makes all of the final decisions and is cognizant of the risks inherent in not following a DMC recommendation. In practice, once a DMC uncovers an issue, they generally negotiate a solution with the sponsor. Rarely however would the sponsor refuse to terminate a study after receiving a recommendation from the sponsor. An intermediate step might be to suspend the enrollment of new patients until more information can be gathered by the sponsor's pharmacovigilence staff and the DMC members.

7.2 Decision-Making Environment

Before embarking on the DMC decision-making process, we should describe the context in which DMC decisions on safety and efficacy are made. Schactman and Wittes (2015) contrast the difference in safety analysis at the end of the trial by sponsor staff with the analysis done by DMC members at their closed session meetings. Obviously, the DMC members meet for short sessions only several times per year and do not have the expertise with the intervention that sponsor staff have when they perform their analysis at the end of the trial. Also, at the end of the trial, all the data will be site monitored and cleaned and will be analyzed by sponsor-standard regulatory submission tables. Sponsor staff will be able to better integrate into their analysis laboratory values, concomitant meds, and preexisting and intercurrent disease. DMC members review data that have not yet been cleaned using tables that are developed as the trial continues and must make decisions without any knowledge of efficacy. Moreover, even data that have been cleaned can be changed by an investigator who may rethink MedDRA preferred term or severity.

DMCs make decisions on safety without knowledge of efficacy. Even when DMC members receive some efficacy information during the trial, efficacy is not usually established until the end of the trial. For many nonlife-threatening indications, DMCs will view SAE evidence differently than they would for a less-serious indication.

There are some limitations to considering efficacy data available during the trial. First, there is likely to be insufficient power to detect a treatment difference early in the trial. Second, some DMC members are not specialists in the disease but rather in expected adverse events. The AE experts together with the biostatistician may be uncomfortable making efficacy decisions. For some small DMCs, there may be only one physician on the panel capable of making the decision. This person or persons will often claim that the efficacy endpoints established for the trial are not the way specialists evaluate patient benefit in practice. Metrics such as the SLEDAI in systemic lupus erythematosus (Bombardier, Gladman, Urowitz et al. 1992), PASI score in psoriasis (Fredriksson and Pettersson 1978), the Ritchie score in rheumatoid arthritis (Lewis, O'Sullivan, and Rumfield 1988), and so on, were all developed for cohort evaluation but not for evaluating an individual patient and there are still questions about their appropriateness in clinical trials (Ashcroft, Li Wan Po, Williams et al. 1999). It is true that considerable other patient information may be available but the DMC would have to make a special request to the sponsor for this information and such a request might send a signal to the sponsor that a significant safety issue has arisen.

7.3 Risk versus Benefit Analyses

In Chapter 4, we enumerated the guidances dealing with risk versus benefit issued in the last decade by agencies such as ICH, FDA, CIOMS, and EMA. These documents deal mainly with requirements for periodic reporting of data useful in the risk versus benefit decision.

Even before these guidance documents were issued, sponsors performed some kind of risk versus benefit analysis as part of the regulatory submission. Of course, the objectivity of this analysis can be questioned. The DMC will have limited information to perform such an analysis but one recent example of DMC decision making for risk versus benefit is the gradual discovery of cardiovascular risks in the PERT trial. Wittes, Barrett-Connor, Braunwald et al. (2007) present a detailed history of their collaboration and risk versus benefit decision to terminate the trail. In the United Kingdom, the National Institute of Health and Clinical Excellence (NICE) does perform these analyses after drug approval in the United Kingdom (U.K. National Health Service 2008) and the German Institute for Quality and Efficiency in Health Care (IQWiG) provides similar analyses as part of the German drug approval process (German Institute for Quality and Efficiency in Health Care 2008). Many factors are involved in such an analysis and a detailed analysis is beyond the scope of a DMC. Most often, risk versus benefit analysis are done only after considerable postmarket experience with a drug such as by Siu and Rowinsky (1998) for irinotecan in solid tumors, by Ziemssen, Neuhaus, and Hohlfield (2001) for glatiramer acetate in multiple sclerosis, Mikuls and Moreland (2003) for infliximab in rheumatoid arthritis, and Cranney and Adachi (2005) for raloxifene in postmenopausal osteoporosis.

For quantification of benefit versus risk, Xia and Jiang (2014) conclude that although many metrics have been proposed for risk versus benefit (see, e.g., Chuang-Stein, Entsuah, and Pritchett 2008; Guo, Pandey, Doyle et al. 2010; Ke,

Jiang, and Snapinn 2015), none has emerged as satisfactory under all conditions and qualitative expert judgment appears to be the best approach to date.

Indeed, no single qualitative methodology is employed in the assessment of risk versus benefit. Risk versus benefit analysis is an important and evolving field.

Much of formal risk versus benefit analysis lies in the hands of the sponsors and the investigators who will write a final manuscript on the trial. There is one "quick and dirty" risk versus benefit assessment that DMC members can perform during closed sessions—calculation of number needed to treat (NNT), number needed to harm (NNH), and the NNH/NNT ratio.

The *number needed to treat (NNT)* calculation was described by Laupacis, Sackett, and Roberts (1988). In a two-arm clinical trial, let group 1 represent the control group and group 2 denote the experimental group. Then

$$NNT = \frac{1}{p_1 - p_2}$$

where
p_1 = unfavorable event rate in the control group
p_2 = unfavorable event rate in the experimental group

The number needed to harm (NNH) is computed as

$$NNH = \frac{1}{q_2 - q_1}$$

where
q_1 = adverse event rate in the control group
q_2 = adverse event rate in the experimental group

The NNT is interpreted as the number of patients that would have to be treated with the experimental treatment to prevent an additional unfavorable event (death, disease progression, nonresponse, etc.) compared to control treatment. The NNH is interpreted as how many patients would have to be treated with the experimental treatment to observe an additional adverse event compared to control treatment. Now, the ratio RB = NNH/NNT represents the number of unfavorable events that are prevented by the experimental treatment for each AE caused. NNT and NNH can be calculated using MedCalc (2016a).

This calculation can be illustrated with an example. The ALTTO trial was an adjuvant breast cancer randomized phase III trial with four treatment groups representing different strategies for lapatinib and/or trastuzumab with primary efficacy endpoint disease-free survival (DFS)

(Piccart-Gebhart, Holmes, Baselga et al. 2016). Investigators were concerned about the grade 3 + 4 diarrhea adverse event. Table 7.1 displays the relevant risk–benefit data for two treatment groups that we will use for illustration T (trastuzumab alone, control) and L + T (lapatinib plus trastuzumab, experimental). The efficacy (proportion of recurrences/deaths at 4 years) and safety (proportion with grade 3 + 4 diarrhea) are shown. The efficacy proportions were calculated as 1 – the DFS reading on the Kaplan–Meier curve. Carrying out the calculations, we see the NNT at 50 meaning that we would have to treat 50 patients on L + T to prevent an additional recurrence compared to T. The NNH is computed at 7.14 meaning that we would treat about 7 patients on L + T to observe an additional grade 3 + 4 diarrhea over T. The NNH/NNT ratio is 0.143. A ratio greater than one would be an indication of preference for L + T and this was not observed here. This makes sense with the considerable AE diarrhea burden of L + T and essentially no advantage in efficacy. It is ratios of less than one that DMC members would be looking for if they make these quick and dirty calculations during the closed session. The two biostatisticians in the room would be logical people to lead such a discussion. DMC members might be directed to the website www.thennt.com where NNT and NNH values for some common interventions are presented. This might provide a context for assessing the level of RB ratio observed in the trial. Of course, the use of this metric is more complicated. It would ideally be exposure corrected and be observed over time. Calculation of confidence intervals would also be useful but more sophistication over our example would be overkill for use in DMC meetings where the ratio would be used just to begin a clinical discussion. Ke, Jiang, and Snapinn (2015) discuss the analytic extensions to NNH/NNT.

TABLE 7.1

Risk and Benefit Data from the ALTTO Clinical Trial

Group	T Group 1, Control	L + T Group 2, Experimental
N	2076	2061
Proportion with recurrence or death at 4 years	0.14 (p_1)	0.12 (p_2)
NNT (number needed to treat)	50	
Proportion with grade 3 + 4 diarrhea	0.13 (q_1)	0.153 (q_2)
NNH (number needed to harm)	7.14	
RB = NNH/NNT (risk–benefit ratio)	0.143	

Source: Piccart-Gebhart, M. et al. 2016. *Journal of Clinical Oncology,* **34**, 1034–1042.
Note: L = lapatinib, T = trastuzumab.

7.4 When a Safety Issue Arises

We now come to the point where a DMC has found an SAE that appears to occur more in the experimental group than the control group and they feel that what they know about efficacy will not overcome this differential. This discussion assumes that the confirmatory trial in question has only one experimental arm. Clearly if there is more than one experimental arm representing different doses, schedules, formulations, and so on, safety actions can be taken on only certain experimental treatment groups, and not necessarily all groups. How does the DMC proceed for a single experimental group? First, statistical significance is neither necessary nor sufficient for a DMC to take action. Statistical significance is a function of power of the statistical tests used and, of course, it is vulnerable to multiplicity and the unplanned use of formal statistical inference for the SAE. The experimental treatment might have only a slightly higher incidence of a life-threatening cardiovascular SAE than the active control but if the drug will eventually be marketed to hundreds of thousands of patients that will translate into so many more potential public health problems that it may be unethical to continue to expose the clinical trial subjects to this drug. Of course, the DMC members will be reading case narratives and, perhaps, requesting further information. The discussion around narratives—predisposing conditions, function of age and gender, and concomitant medications, will often generate possible alternative explanations for the observed SAEs.

DMCs often face the question of how long they should wait until they inform the sponsor of the safety issue. This depends on the individual circumstances of the SAE, indication, and other aspects of the drug's safety profile. A calculation of conditional power as described later in this chapter might be useful here. Further discussion of this matter will be found below under "Trial Termination."

When a safety issue arises through the DMC's review of safety data, a number of activities can take place ranging from unmasking to trial termination. A summary is presented in ascending order in Table 7.2.

7.4.1 Unmasking

In many cases, the DMC will be unmasked either by plan or de facto. In some cases, the DMC will be partially unmasked and a decision may be made to identify what the group symbols (A, B or Blue, Green, etc.) represent. Alternatively if there are, say, seven patients who have an SAE of some concern and the split is 1 versus 6 or 0 versus 7, the DMC may seek further information including the identification of the groups. This method neither reveals the treatments of the individual patients nor the group identities. Even if the DMC requests treatment assignments of the seven patients, they have learned only the assignment of those patients. Many DMCs think all

TABLE 7.2

Possible Actions to Be Taken by a DMC after Observing an SAE of Concern (Listed in Ascending Order of Trial Impact)

Action	Description	Comments
Unmasking	Identification of treatment groups for the entire cohort or just for patients with the SAE.	This is only a transaction between DMC and DAC statistician in the closed session. No sponsor involvement.
"Dear Investigator" letter	DMC recommends that sponsor writes a letter to investigators asking them to beware of SAE signs and symptoms and, where appropriate, suggestions for prevention of the SAE.	There are certain cultural implications in multinational trials where suggestions for medical practice and/or prevention are given in the letter.
Modification of informed consent	DMC recommends to sponsor that specific wording of the SAE be included in a modified informed consent.	Sponsor can only recommend changes to informed consent to investigators. It is up to the investigators and their IRBs to implement. Reconsenting for all patients is recommended over just reconsenting of new patients.
Protocol modification	DMC recommends that protocol be modified for dose, schedule, eligibility, and so on.	DMC must be assertive about the change, sponsor may want to wait until other modifications accumulate and make all changes at one.
Trial termination	After waiting sufficient time for accumulation of further evidence DMC recommends trial termination.	DMC should view this recommendation as the beginning of a dialog with sponsor. Sponsor may have further information about the SAEs and/or other options.

of this as a waste of time and prefer to be just unmasked from the start of the trial. As was said earlier, masking usually begs DMC members to guess treatment assignment, which they usually do correctly, but when wrong, it can create havoc with their decisions for the rest of the trial.

If a DMC is masked and the committee has decided to unmask treatment assignment for those patients who experienced a particular AE, the DMC Chair should first lead the committee through a *decision matrix*. The latter would be what action that committee would take for each possible outcome of the unmasking. If the committee cannot agree on an action there may be no reason for unmasking. Table 7.3 indicates possible actions that might be taken in the case of seven SAEs. Actual actions would depend on the individual trial.

7.4.2 "Dear Investigator" Letter

The DMC may feel that it is sufficient at this point to recommend that the sponsor sends a *"Dear Investigator" letter* to each investigator informing them

TABLE 7.3

Hypothetical Decision Matrix for Seven Patients Reporting an SAE of Concern

Frequency of SAE by Treatment Group		
A	B	Action
0	7	Request the identity of A, B. If B is experimental, begin the discussion of ascending decisions as in Table 7.1. If control is active discuss if expected. If not, search for more information on active control drug.
1	6	Same as 0–7 above
2	5	Same as 0–7 above
3	4	No action
4	3	No action
5	2	Same as 0–7 above with roles of A, B reversed
6	1	Same as 5–2 above
7	0	Same as 5–2 above

to watch for signs of the SAE and to inform patients to contact the investigator if they experience symptoms related to this SAE. The letter may also contain suggestions for preventing the SAE if, for example, the SAE was a postsurgical infection. The wording here must be diplomatic because it can be taken by some investigators as insulting. Something like a postsurgical infection in a global trial brings up many differentials in training, practice of medicine, and supervision. Although the letter may be aimed at certain countries it must go to all investigators. A request for a "Dear Investigator" letter is usually accompanied by a request that the sponsor's clinical research associates enforce the letter through on-site discussion with investigator and staff and follow-up auditing. At future meetings, the DMC should inform the DAC that they would like to see a pre-post letter analysis of change in incidence. If there is not a reduction in incidence as a result of the letter further action may be taken.

The DMC will usually ask the sponsor to draft the "Dear Investigator" letter for comment by the DMC before sending.

7.4.3 Modification of Informed Consent

The DMC may request a rewording of the informed consent form adding a warning to patients of the SAE of concern. The sponsor may send out a suggested rewording but each investigator site has the right to word the modification in their own way and negotiate the change with their IRB or ethics committee. When a modification of informed consent occurs, the question of reconsenting patients already in the trial arises. It is not considered good practice to show the modified consent form only to new patients entering the trial. Patients may be asked to sign the modified consent form at their next clinic visit. An alternative is to call back all patients regardless of the date of the next clinic visit for their review and signing of the informed consent document. This should be done only in the most extreme cases where the SAE is life-threatening and the patients are taking oral medication. In protocols where patients are dosed only through injections or infusions at the clinic, calling in patients for review would be unnecessary. Many investigator staffs are communicating with their patients through websites and/ or e-mail. Hence, it is possible to make patients, or their family members/ caregivers, aware of a new SAE prior to their coming into the clinic. It is possible that some patients will refuse to sign the modified informed consent and drop out of the trial. This is their right. That this, or reduced compliance to oral medication, might be a consequence of reconsenting should not be part of the decision of whether or not to reconsent.

7.4.4 Protocol Modification

The DMC may feel that the presence of certain SAEs indicates that a protocol modification is in order—change in dosage/schedule, eligibility, and so on. Sponsors will often reply that, due to the long process of running the revised protocol through all IRBs involved, they prefer to wait until enough changes come about from other sources and make the change all at once. The DMC must be prepared to indicate that the time for change is now if they feel that patients are at risk.

7.4.5 Trial Termination

A recommendation of trial termination usually does not come at the first sign of a disturbing SAE treatment difference. What appears to be a disturbing treatment difference early in the trial could be a random occurrence that will correct itself in time. In time-to-event analyses, it could be a manifestation of the "bad news travels first" phenomenon. In this scenario, SAEs are reported as soon as they occur but before reports of follow-up time for the many patients not experiencing these events. Hence, the analysis has an overrepresentation of events compared to exposure. The DMC may request another analysis of an appropriate subset of the routine analysis before the next scheduled meeting. This ad hoc meeting will usually be covered by teleconference but, in some cases, the DMC may feel it necessary to meet face-to-face to go over enhanced and updated narratives and other information apart from statistical reports that the DMC may have requested previously. It is important for the DMC to take turnaround time into account when requesting ad hoc reports from the DAC (see *DMCounselor*, Q7.5 below).

If the DMC feels that trial termination is a viable option, it should take this as the beginning of a dialog with the sponsor where the DMC presents this as their pending decision. This conversation would usually be with the sponsor's pharmacovigilance unit rather than the protocol team. This will keep the latter properly masked while discussions proceed. As was mentioned above, the pharmacovigilance unit might first offer to stop enrollment of new patients on the trial while discussions and analysis continue. The pharmacovigilance staff may have information about the drug or the SAEs that the DMC has not considered. The DMC should not be intimidated by responses from the sponsor but should definitely listen to the points to be made.

The sponsor will ask the DMC if they have considered the overall benefit as well as risk. The issues involved in risk versus benefit have been discussed above. The relevance of taking that matter up will depend on the indication and the nature of the SAE. In oncology and congestive heart failure trials, more risk may be taken if there is some evidence of benefit or at least a feeling that there is no reason to doubt the hypothesized benefit and the latter would outweigh the harm. In trials of seasonal rhinitis or skin rash, there may be less tolerance for SAEs especially with effective drugs already on the market with a more favorable safety profile.

For many indications, deaths and SAEs may be considered by the sponsor to be part of the disease process. If there is an excess of these events in the control group, the sponsor may argue that this is not a safety issue at all but early evidence of efficacy. The sponsor may hesitate to terminate the trial early because of uncertainty if the regulatory agencies would accept the curtailed trial as evidence worthy of drug approval. On ethical grounds, the sponsor may indicate that the control group patients are at no greater risk than any person who has the disease under investigation not participating in the trial. While this defense is reasonable, the DMC may want the sponsor to at least set a stopping rule by which they would indicate how much of an imbalance would not be acceptable. This stopping rule would have to be discussed with the regulatory agencies to determine how the trial could be salvaged if it had to be terminated according to this rule. In cases like this and similar cases, it should be clinical and ethical issues that determine the course of action and not the result of a statistical hypothesis test.

The DMC must understand the financial implications of their decision and expect there to be tension in these deliberations. In certain regions of the world, the risk versus benefit decision in the presence of an SAE may be different than would be the case in North America or Western Europe and DMCs should be aware of these distinctions. After this exchange, the DMC must move swiftly to make their final decision on termination or to arrange another decision point in the near term. The future decision point should only come about because of further information to be obtained by the sponsor that the DMC considers relevant.

Should the DMC make a recommendation for termination, the sponsor will decide whether or not to accept the recommendation. Trial termination will follow immediately in most cases. If the trial is to be terminated, a decision must be made about possible continuation of patients currently on the experimental arm who are tolerating the drug and receiving benefit. The sponsor may either terminate the trial for all patients or leave the decision of continuation up to each investigator and their patient to decide. Any patient who continues will have to be reconsented.

In making an important decision such as trial termination, it is important that the DMC report to the same person(s) they normally report to after a DMC meeting. If they are to report to a senior officer of the sponsor if termination is recommended and the sponsor team otherwise, an awkward situation occurs when the DMC Chair tells the sponsor team that he/she cannot reveal the outcome of the meeting but rather must contact the senior officer. Rumors will spread through the company very quickly in this case. If a senior officer wants to be the first to know of trial termination or other important decision, then, he/she must be the person to contact after routine meetings as well.

7.4.6 Unmasking the Sponsor

All of the responses to SAEs of concern described above have the potential of unmasking the sponsor. If the DMC is itself masked, the sponsor would not necessarily be unmasked in being asked to write a "Dear Investigator" letter, modify informed consent, and so on. If it is known that the DMC is unmasked, this would be a signal to the sponsor that most patients with a particular SAE are on the experimental treatment arm. However, this is not a major problem because this information is limited to a few patients and the sponsor would have these clues anyway in observing SAEs expected to occur on the experimental arm. Prior to contacting the sponsor, the DMC must decide on a wording of the recommendation that will minimize unmasking the sponsor. It is usually the DMC Chair who would have the responsibility of contacting the sponsor and providing the recommendation. Upon hearing the decision, the sponsor will usually assume that the DMC has observed a treatment difference that has motivated this change. The DMC should not reveal whether or not they have unmasked and should not provide more information other than we think the following steps are in order. Statements like "the DMC feels that a "Dear Investigator" letter is in order" or "the DMC is recommending a protocol modification" are sufficient.

7.5 Information beyond the Present Trial

The DMC may utilize safety evidence from other trials as part of their decision-making process. For data from the same drug, the sources of information would be in the investigator brochure issued by the sponsor. However, more detail may be required than what initially appears in this document.

The question arises should the DMC seek data from other drugs and other indications. It is not the DMC's job to review data from other trials but, when important safety decisions must be made, it is not the DMC's job to ignore such data either. A committee concerned with serious adverse events on a trial of rofecoxib (Baron, Sandler, Bresalier et al. 2006) might choose to seek data on the related drug celecoxib (Lee, Ji, and Song 2007). Similarly, a revelation of a postmarket safety issue for diabetes drugs rosiglitazone and pioglitazone (Devchand 2008) might trigger some extra vigilance by a DMC for a clinical trial for muraglitazar (Nissen, Wolski, and Topol 2005) for the same indication. The committee may seek data from other indications of the same drug. A DMC meeting on rituximab for rheumatoid arthritis (Cohen, Emery, Greenwald et al. 2006) review data previously collected on rituximab in non-Hodgkin's lymphoma (van Oers, Klasa, Marcus et al. 2006) beyond what might be in the investigator brochure. Although the open label extension studies are not controlled trials, DMC members might want to search these studies for further consideration of AEs that arise in the controlled confirmatory trial. In seeking data from other trials, the DMC must seek data trials that are contemporaneous with their trial. As Ioannidis, Mulrow, and Goodman (2006) point out, more recent trials may use new technologies to assess adverse events such as endoscopy for gastrointestinal bleeding versus the previous method of clinical evaluation. They also caution that trials of drugs used in the past may have low discontinuation rates due to AEs because there were no or fewer alternative treatments at that time. The current trial may have higher discontinuation rates because of the availability of more alternative treatments. The older trial might have higher AE rates than the current trial due to longer exposure because fewer alternative treatments were available at the time. Also, differentials in frequency and timing of follow-up visits might affect between-trial differences in the level of adverse events reported. Table 7.4 presents a summary of cautions

TABLE 7.4

Cautions about Using Data from Previous Clinical Trials of Same or Similar Drugs to Compare with Data in Current Trial

1. Previous trials may have had different eligibility requirements and may have allowed different concomitant medications
2. Current trial may use newer techniques for finding AEs (e.g., endoscopy, CT scans) or newer adverse event dictionaries (e.g., MedDRA)
3. Drugs used in the past may have low discontinuation rates due to fewer alternative treatments than the present drug or may have higher AE rates due to longer exposure because of fewer alternatives
4. Differences in frequency and timing of follow-up visits between trials
5. Differences in the use of spontaneous or solicited adverse event reporting

in using data from previous trials in DMC decisions. For clinical trials that enroll normal healthy volunteers, such as infectious disease vaccine trials, some DMCs may consider comparing SAEs such as trial death rates with those from vital statistics. Here again there are cautions about comparability. Clinical trial populations are expected to be healthier than the general population because these subjects are healthy enough to make the regular visits required by the trial and because, as trial participants, they are being examined and followed by clinicians more frequently than those of the same age–gender group in the general population.

In recent years, there has been an increasing use of databases and registries to investigate drug safety issues. FDA has had its MedWatch voluntary reporting program for some time (U.S. Food and Drug Administration 2008a), they are now working with the health insurance industry to build the Sentinel database (U.S. Food and Drug Administration 2010), and the American Society for Clinical Oncology recently launched its CancerLinq database which is pooling cancer treatment records from oncologists all over the world (Schilsky, Michels, Kearbey et al. 2014; Shah, Stewart, Kolacevski et al. 2016). Ryan, Madigan, and Schuemie (2015) review the state of the art in using observational data in pharmacovigilence. Gibbons and Amatya (2016) review the issues and describe statistical methods for analysis of spontaneous AE reports and use of medical claims data for drug safety research.

Traditionally outside data would come into play only when an important safety decision must be made and where members felt that an extra comfort level from additional data was necessary before a decision could be made. However, the FDA has now issued a draft guidance suggesting that sponsors create safety assessment committees (SAC) to continuously review the safety profile of a drug in development and drive the task of incorporating data from other trials of this drug or similar drugs, epidemiologic studies, animal studies, and so on, to decide if an observed adverse event must be reported as serious (U.S. Food and Drug Administration 2015a). The objective of this guidance is to enable recognition of serious adverse events earlier than just using accumulating data from a single trial. It is not likely that the DMC would also serve as an SAC since it is best for the DMC to concentrate on one trial. The SAC may consist of outside experts as well as sponsor representatives. Already, Gould and Wang (2016) and Schnell and Ball (2016) have developed Bayesian methods to perform SAE monitoring on blinded trials using prior information from other sources. Once the SAC proposal is implemented and Bayesian methods such as these are further developed, DMCs are likely to be in periodic communication with the SAC, perhaps even with a common member to discuss the global picture of SAEs associated with a specific experimental treatment. While this is a good model, it is not clear how the limited staff of an Infant Pharma sponsor could keep track of both a DMC and an SAC or to have the finances to pay for such an operation.

7.6 Meta-Analysis

Closely related to the issue of utilizing data outside the trial is the use of the statistical method of *meta-analysis* (Whitehead 2002). The classic definition of meta-analysis is "the statistical analysis of a large collection of analysis results from individual studies for the purpose of integrating the findings" (Glass 1976). The SPERT report (Crowe, Xia, Berlin et al. 2009) indicated that meta-analysis of safety might be useful in safety analysis and CIOMS IV (Council for International Organizations of Medical Sciences 2005) indicates that meta-analysis should be a routine part of the drug development process and warns that crude pooling of data across trials should be avoided. Hence, it is possible that DMCs may be provided with sponsor-generated meta-analyses.

In response to a controversy over cardiovascular risk among Type II diabetes mellitus patients treated with rosiglitazone (Nissen and Wolski 2007), the FDA issued a guidance calling for all Type II diabetes clinical trial protocols to provide statistical evidence that the sample size for the trial is sufficient to detect cardiovascular effects (U.S. Food and Drug Administration 2008b). Ibrahim, Chen, Xia et al. (2012) subsequently proposed using Bayesian meta-analysis to assess the adequacy of a diabetes drug development clinical program to evaluate cardiovascular risk. The method employs Bayesian borrowing to incorporate data from clinical trials outside the current development program.

In the clinical trials context, meta-analysis entails either obtaining summary data from published trials or the raw individual-level data from previous trials. Then, sophisticated statistical methods are used to integrate the data across trials to get combined estimates of efficacy or safety.

A DMC might be presented a meta-analysis by a sponsor or request that one be created to augment a safety analysis. The reasons for this could be that safety data exist on other trials within this clinical program or elsewhere for other indications of the experimental drug. Besides, a more precise estimate of AE incidence meta-analysis might permit subgroup analyses that are not possible with the data from the current trial. The sponsor, or preferably an independent group, might perform a meta-analysis when a serious safety concern arises indicating that this occurrence is a chance outlier and a meta-analysis would provide a more realistic estimate. DMCs might see meta-analyses produced by the sponsor if they are reviewing the integrated summary of safety. Here, the sponsor might use meta-analysis to refine the dose–response relationship or to see how an overall safety effect might hold among subgroups of patients.

The first consideration in reviewing a meta-analysis is whether it is based on *aggregate patient data (APD)* or *individual patient data (IPD)*. An APD meta-analysis is performed on data extracted from the literature. An IPD meta-analysis is performed on the actual raw patient-level data from the various studies. APD meta-analysis is highly vulnerable to the *publication bias*. The results of negative trials might never be published and those trials might have had an unfavorable safety profile for the experimental drug. The data needed for analysis may not be available from all trials or not in the same format. For example, adverse events might be defined differently, age groups might be presented in different intervals, and so on. The definitions needed on adverse event classification and severity might not be included in the publications.

Many of these issues exist for IPD meta-analysis as well. The issues in using data from outside the trial summarized in the previous section and in Table 7.4 apply to meta-analysis as well. DMC members should ask the sponsor if they prepared a meta-analysis protocol before embarking on the analysis where the preanalysis procedures for publication selection, trial qualification, and so on, should be described.

Berlin (2008) discusses several additional issues in the use of meta-analysis in safety assessment. He is concerned that meta-analyses might confound dose and indication. An antiepileptic drug might be used at a lower dose for migraines than for epilepsy. Combining these data might lead to misleading results. If dose differs by gender, researchers must make sure that dose–gender data for the required AEs are available in the literature or in all prospective trials under consideration. It would be important to determine if any of the trials being combined have an active control and if the active control is the same across these trials. A case has been made previously for reporting patient years of follow-up in all trials. Will these data be available in all trials under consideration?

Meta-analysis can be done with the treatment difference being estimated considered *fixed* or varying in a *random* manner across trials (DerSimonian and Laird 1986). A test of heterogeneity across trials would be useful in making this decision and the sponsor should provide these results. Random effects models introduce an extra source of variation which might make it more difficult to find a statistically significant treatment difference in AE incidence. The choice between fixed and random should be justified by the sponsor. Tests of sensitivity to assumptions are helpful to see the extent that conclusions are influenced by classifications, trial inclusions/exclusions, fixed/random, and so on. Berlin, Crowe, Whalen et al. (2013) provide further practical advice on the use of meta-analysis in drug safety. They remind the reader that a key issue in reaching conclusions in meta-analyses is whether the differences among studies are merely due to pure random error (statistical heterogeneity) or due to an assignable cause—clinical heterogeneity (differences in patient characteristics due to eligibility or geographic region, dose/schedule) or methodological heterogeneity (study design, masking policy).

Indeed, still another researcher group has created the *PRISMA statement (Preferred Reporting Items for Systematic Reviews and Meta-Analysis)*. The PRISMA criteria provide a checklist of items that should be included in a meta-analysis report. They do not attach weights to the individual items but

TABLE 7.5

Checklist for the Review of Meta-Analyses of Safety Data across Clinical Trials

1. What are the stated objectives of the meta-analysis?
2. Was the meta-analysis prepared by sponsor staff or an independent organization?
3. Was a preanalysis meta-analysis protocol prepared stating how publications and trials were selected, methods of analysis, and so on?
4. For retrospective meta-analysis:
   a. How were publications selected?
   b. Is there reason to suspect publication bias?
   c. Can the extent of bias be estimated in some way?
5. All issues in Table 7.4 above apply to the review of meta-analyses.
6. By what criteria did trials qualify for inclusion?
7. Evaluate the extent of compliance with the PRISMA criteria.
8. What trials were considered but excluded from analysis? For what reasons?
9. How are adverse events classified and graded across trials?
10. Are doses and indications being combined?
11. Do some of the trials use active controls? Are they the same active controls across trials?
12. Was a test of heterogeneity performed? What are the results? What are the clinical, methodological, and statistical heterogeneity considerations?
13. Which factors are considered fixed and which are considered random? What is the justification for this decision?
14. Were tests of sensitivity done to see if there is consistency in conclusions across different definitions of inclusion, fixed/random, and so on?

DMC members might want to refer to this list in evaluating meta-analyses that are presented to them. The PRISMA list can be found in Liberati, Altman, Tetzlaff et al. (2009) as well as in Hammad, Neyarapally, Pinhiero et al. (2013). The latter review recent published meta-analyses to assess the compliance with the PRISMA standards and found mixed results.

Table 7.5 presents a checklist of items DMC members might consider in reviewing meta-analyses of safety data across clinical trials.

7.7 Planned Interim Analyses Regarding Efficacy

This book concentrates on DMC safety responsibilities. However, confirmatory trial protocols call for an interim analysis where the trial can be terminated due to early evidence of efficacy, terminated due to futility as described above, continued with the same sample size originally specified in the protocol, or continued with an increased sample size. The interim analysis will take place in closed session and will be run by both the DAC biostatistician who produced the analysis necessary for the meeting and by the biostatistical member of the DMC. This section will present some of the rationale and frequentist statistical thinking that goes into these analyses.

In Chapter 5, we defined Type I error as the probability that we reject the null hypothesis of no treatment effect when it is true. We also called this regulator risk because regulators would not want a product that did not have efficacy to appear to be effective and possibly enter the market. Type II error is the probability that we accept the null hypothesis when it is false, that is, declare a product not to be effective when, in fact, there is evidence of efficacy. This is appropriately called sponsor risk.

We have already described the frequentist conundrum over multiplicity in Chapter 5—the notion that repeatedly testing a hypothesis increasing the Type I (regulator) error. We might want to test the efficacy hypothesis at some midpoint in the trial under the justification that early termination in the face of overwhelming evidence of efficacy it would be unethical to continue to expose patients to the inferior control treatment. Here, the multiple testing would raise Type I error. To prevent inflation of Type I error, statisticians have developed *group sequential designs* that allow for an interim test of the null hypothesis leading to possible early termination of the trial for superiority while preserving the overall Type I error. These designs are also referred to as *"alpha spending functions"* because Type I error is often called alpha error. Two closely related group sequential methods are *O'Brien–Fleming* (O'Brien and Fleming 1979) and *Lan–DeMets* (Lan and DeMets 1983). A review of methods of interim analysis sometimes referred to as statistical monitoring can be found in Proschan, Lan, and Wittes (2006).

Interim analyses also offer the opportunity to test for *futility*, that is, an assessment of how likely are we to reject the null hypothesis at the trial given some assumptions of *"drift"* or trajectory of future efficacy results. The futility method most often seen by DMCs is conditional power. A review of methods and rationale for futility analysis in clinical trials is given by Herson, Buyse, and Wittes (2012). We will see an example of a futility analysis later in this chapter.

Protocols sometimes specify a sample size reestimation at the time of interim analysis. This is prudent because often, the initial assumptions regarding variability are wrong resulting in a smaller sample size than necessary. We will discuss sample size reestimation in Chapter 8 under adaptive designs.

We now turn to Table 7.6 for a hypothetical example of a rheumatoid arthritis trial to describe the group sequential and futility analyses as the DMC would likely see them.

The primary clinical endpoint for this trial is ACR-N AUC, and percent difference from baseline to 24 weeks. This is the area under the curve of serial measurements of ACR-N which is described in Bathon, Martin, Fleischmann et al. (2000) and is expressed in units percent-years. There are two groups—control and experimental. The null hypothesis on Delta (the difference between groups) is zero, and the alternative hypothesis for Delta is 4.5. Assuming a common standard deviation of 14, and specifying a significance level (Type I error) of 0.05 and a power of 0.90, we can derive the required sample size in each group as 205. We now want to build into the design of this trial an interim analysis halfway through the trial or

TABLE 7.6

Interim Analysis of Efficacy: Hypothetical Rheumatoid Arthritis Trial

Clinical Endpoint	ACR-N AUC Percent Difference from Baseline to 24 Weeks (Pct Years)	
	Group 1 (Control)	Group 2 (Experimental)
Null hypothesis for difference between Groups 1 and 2 (Delta)	0	
Alternate hypothesis for difference between Groups 1 and 2	4.5	
Common standard deviation (SD)	14	
Significance level/power	0.05/0.90	
Total N required	205	205
O'Brien–Fleming significance levels:		
At information time = 0.05	0.003	
At final analysis (information time—1.0)	0.048	
N at interim analysis (information time = 0.5)	102	104
SD at interim	12.2	12.5
Observed Delta	1.4	
Attained significance level	0.180	
Decision	Continue the trial	
Nonbinding futility analysis at interim Conditional power:		
Assume null hypothesis drift (Diff = 0)	0.025	
Assume current results drift (Diff = 1.7)	0.120	
Assume alternate hypothesis drift (Diff = 4.5)	0.740	
Decision regarding futility	Nonbinding futility	

when half the patients have completed the trial or at *information time* 0.5. It is important to note here that in time-to-event trials (overall survival [OS], progression-free survival [PFS]), the denominator of information time is not the total number of patients but the total number of events. Anyway, the DAC can calculate that the O'Brien–Fleming boundary for an interim analysis at information time 0.5 is significance level 0.003. This means we can only terminate this trial early for superiority of the experimental treatment if the attained significance level is less than 0.003. In order to maintain an overall Type I error of 0.05 hypothesis test at the end of the trial will use the critical value 0.048. It makes sense that the early stopping boundary of 0.003 be so low because we would only want to stop early if the evidence were overwhelming. Of course, there are reasons that we might not want to terminate early even with this evidence. To continue to the end might provide more persuasive evidence to the medical community and would certainly provide more safety data to the DMC and regulators. In any case in our hypothetical example at sample sizes 102 and 104 with standard deviations as shown, we observe a Delta of 1.4 with an attained significance level of 0.180 so that there is no evidence for early termination.

Sequential analysis of safety data is rarely done but Ball, Piller, and Silverman (2011) have developed a Bayesian method for continuous safety monitoring of blinded data. This analysis is done parallel to efficacy analysis and would, presumably, concentrate on Tier 1 (AESI) adverse events.

DMC members might encounter an ad hoc alpha-spending function known as the *Haybittle–Peto* alpha spending (Haybittle 1971). Under this plan, researchers spend Type I error of 0.001 at some point in the trial and can still test the hypothesis at the end of the trial at the usual 0.05 significance level. This is because, although there is a correction for multiplicity, the final significance level is easily rounded to 0.05. Haybittle–Peto is generally used when there is an accidental unmasking or when the sponsor has a separate unit perform data cleaning during the trial. There is no formal hypothesis test at the 0.001 level but taking the "hit" of 0.001 usually satisfies regulators.

As stated above, early termination even with evidence of superiority is not always prudent and, hence, DMCs can expect to see futility analyses at interim more frequently than group sequential tests for early termination due to superiority. We should never use the term "futility analysis" without the modifier *binding* or *nonbinding*. A binding futility analysis means that the sponsor has decided before the interim analysis takes place that the trial will terminate if the futility condition is reached. Conversely, a nonbinding futility analysis means the DMC can advise not to terminate when a futility boundary is crossed and, regardless, the sponsor can continue the trial in that situation.

Using the conditional power method of assessing futility, we compute the power to reject the null hypothesis at the end of the trial under three "drift" assumptions—(1) that the null hypothesis of no difference prevails for the rest of the trial, (2) that the current treatment difference prevails for the rest of the trial, and (3) that the alternate hypothesis Delta (4.5) prevails for the rest of the trial. We see that even if the alternate hypothesis of as large as 4.5 prevailed, we would only have a power of 0.740 to reject at the end. Most DMCs and sponsors would want a higher conditional power than 0.740 to continue especially since it is unlikely that the alternative would prevail. Under the current trend, the probability for rejection at the end of the trial is only 0.120. Thus, the DMC might advise the sponsor that futility has been reached. Note that this hypothetical trial specified a nonbinding futility analysis.

Now that the ball is in the sponsor's court, their team will have to make a decision on what to do next. Herson, Buyse, and Wittes (2012) discuss this decision point in detail. The reasons to terminate would include an unfavorable safety profile, even secondary endpoints are showing negative signs, competing therapies are having much better outcomes, and sponsor money can be better spent elsewhere. Surprising to some, there are many reasons the sponsor might want to continue the trial in spite of the futility calculation—patient characteristics might change in the latter part of the trial bringing patients with better prognostic factors into the trial. This usually happens when a competing trial with slightly better eligibility requirements has closed, site monitoring on the trial may have been insufficient to date to have confidence in the data, the data might still permit approval in other countries, and desire to learn more about efficacy in certain subgroups of patients to plan new trials. This underscores the importance for all written and verbal communication of futility analysis in a trial to carry the modifier binding or nonbinding.

In our example, the efficacy variable used for interim analysis is the same as the one to be used for the final analysis. This is common for rheumatoid arthritis trials. For oncology trials where the primary efficacy endpoint is overall survival (OS), it is not uncommon for the interim analysis to be based on progression-free survival (PFS). While it is known that PFS is not considered an ideal surrogate for OS, it at least allows sponsors for an interim analysis that will take place sooner (i.e., accrue more events sooner) than the one based on OS. Owing to the lack of correlation between PFS and OS in many cancers, sponsors might continue the trial if a futility analysis concluded futility based on PFS because of some confidence that the final analysis of OS will still be positive.

While group sequential analysis of efficacy requires adjustment in final significance level (alpha spending), no such adjustment is needed for conditional power futility analysis because Type I error (regulators risk) is not being spent but rather Type II error (sponsors risk). While it is always advisable for conditional power analysis to be planned in the protocol, the DMC should have the right to request such an analysis from the DAC at any time, especially when they see a somewhat unfavorable safety signal and need to assess how likely the trial is to show positive results at the end, that is, will the average patient benefit from the experimental treatment and balance this against the risk for some patients.

The Bayesian analog to conditional power is *predictive power* (Proschan, Lan, and Wittes 2006). The latter is the posterior probability that the null hypothesis of no treatment difference in AE incidence will be rejected at the end of the trial. Its calculation is conditional on the data collected to date and the prior information. While DMCs might be tempted to use predictive power when a safety concern arises, there are many potential biases inherent in choosing a prior distribution when the treatment difference in incidence at the time of the data review meeting is already known. Lan, Hu, and Proschan (2009) describe the relationship between conditional and predictive power.

7.8 Final Meeting

Under the assumption that the trial was not terminated due to safety, we come to DMC decisions at or shortly after the final DMC meeting. The DMC's precise role at this point will be defined by the DMC Charter. The following are described under the assumption that these tasks have been previously granted to the DMC.

In some cases, the DMC will have the responsibility to review the safety data in the submissions to the regulatory agency. Much of this would be review of tables similar to those already reviewed by the DMC. However, the integrated summary of safety will also be included and DMC review is advisable. This section of the submission will summarize experience of the drug over all studies (Fairweather 1996; Weihrauch and Kubler 2002). There should be no surprises here either. The submission will have a description of the DMC, membership, meeting frequency, and so on. The DMC Chair can check that this information is correct. Closely related would be a review of safety slides to be presented at the advisory committee meeting. This meeting will take place after submission of the new drug application but before the regulatory agency must make its decision on approval.

Some DMCs review the proposed wording of safety in the package insert. The regulatory agency staff will attempt to ensure that the important safety information is presented in a form to be useful to practicing physicians but DMC members may want to comment.

Manuscripts on trial results will be prepared and, if specified in the DMC Charter, it will be important that the DMC members review these manuscripts prior to publication. First, it will be important to see that there will be a published paper even when the efficacy results are negative. The issue of *publication bias* is well known (Dickersin, Olson, Rennie et al. 2002; Dickersin and Rennie 2003). Ioannidis and Lau (2002) have written on shortcomings of many clinical trial papers in the literature with regard to reporting of safety results. They are especially critical of papers that do not report safety data at all, minimize safety data when there are positive efficacy results, or report safety as only "medication was well-tolerated." Adverse events are frequently not reported for indications such as the common cold or dry eye because they are not serious and may be mild in nature. This information is useful to clinicians and patients with these indications as the SAEs are to oncology and cardiovascular patients. Ioannidis, Evans, Getzsche et al. (2004) present further recommendations on reporting safety results. A checklist of safety items to look for in a manuscript is presented in Table 7.7.

7.9 Special Problems with Infant Pharma Companies

DMCs must do their job regardless of the size of the trial sponsor. Infant Pharma companies will be especially concerned about the financial

TABLE 7.7

Checklist for Reporting Safety Results in Clinical Trial Manuscripts

1. Mention of safety results in abstract.
2. Were investigators who assessed AEs masked to treatment assignment?
3. Withdrawals due to toxicity and types of AEs that caused withdrawals.
4. Incidence of laboratory-determined toxicity.
5. Safety tables of incidence of all SAEs and those AEs of interest to the community by severity and treatment group. Not just the most frequently occurring AEs.
6. Patient years of follow-up should be reported for each treatment group.
7. Assay sensitivity—what odds ratios or hazard ratios can be detected by sample size.
8. Severity should be reported as well as the severity scale used.
9. Table of rare and unexpected AEs regardless of severity.
10. Was AE collection spontaneous or solicited? What was the frequency of data collection?
11. Avoid broad categories that do not permit clinical interpretation such as "gastrointestinal AEs," and "skin disorders."

implications of trial termination or even protocol modification or "Dear Investigator" letters. When these companies are public and have only one product in development, any action taken by a DMC may be considered material and thus must be reported in a press release as required in the United States by the Securities and Exchange Commission. When companies are private, the sponsor may still be required by their board of directors to report this information to investors. DMCs should not be intimidated by this requirement. The requirement is to protect investors and the DMC exists to protect patient safety. However, the DMC should be aware of this risk and avoid hasty decisions when serving an Infant Pharma company.

7.10 In Conclusion

We have now followed the life cycle of a DMC from concept, creation to final meeting. We have learned a lot about clinical, statistical, and bias issues along the way. However, the pharmaceutical clinical trial arena is constantly changing with new regulations, clinical advances, new statistical methodology, and so on. We will try to apply what we have already learned to some of these emerging issues in the next chapter. Table 7.8 lists some useful items for the Data Review Plan (DRP). The cumulative list of DRP items will be found in Appendix Table A.2. Table 7.9 displays a list of some potential DMC responsibilities arising in this chapter. A complete list of DMC responsibilities will be found in Appendix Table A.3.

TABLE 7.8

Useful Items for the Data Review Plan (DRP)

1. Will there be a formal analysis of risk vs. benefit?
2. Details of the planned interim analysis
   a. Tables and graphs
   b. Statistical methods and boundaries
   c. Early termination for efficacy
   d. Early termination for futility (binding or nonbinding)
   e. Conditional power analysis
   f. Sample size reestimation

Note: A complete list of DRP items will be found in Appendix Table A.2.

TABLE 7.9

Potential DMC Responsibilities Arising in This Chapter

Suggest and approve "Dear Investigator" letter
Perform "quick and dirty" risk–benefit analysis when appropriate
Contact the unmasked sponsor individual or team on safety concerns
Decision on trial continuation or termination
Use data from outside trial with caution
Conduct planned interim analysis
Request conditional power analysis when needed
In futility analysis enforce "binding" or "nonbinding" as indicated in the protocol and DRP

Note: A complete list of DMC responsibilities will be found in Appendix Table A.3.

DMCounselor

Q7.1 I am sitting on a DMC where the accrual is very slow and is not likely to ever reach the sample size to establish efficacy that appears in the protocol. Can the DMC terminate the trial on the basis that patients are being exposed to a drug where we are not likely to ever learn about its efficacy?

A The answer to this question is "yes" but the DMC must first work with the sponsor on analyzing the reasons for poor accrual, suggest new investigators, change in eligibility requirements, and so on. The DMC and the sponsor should come to an agreement of how long to wait for accrual to improve before the trial is terminated. The more severe and serious the AEs reported the shorter should be the waiting time. While waiting for improvement, you might ask the DAC statistician to make a conditional power or predictive power calculation. This might guide a decision later but this should not be thought of as a strictly statistical issue.

Q7.2 I am serving on a DMC where the active control was approved only a year ago. With unmasking, we are seeing an excess of SAEs in the control group. Can we terminate the trial because of safety issues in the control group?

A The answer is "yes." The DMC exists to protect patient safety regardless of what treatment arm they were assigned. The DMC may not have to terminate the trial. The members can work with the sponsor to choose another active control and, if an ethical alternative exists. This should be done as soon as possible. Many SAEs do not present themselves until postmarket so this situation is not unusual. The DMC should make sure that these control group SAEs are reported to *MedWatch* (U.S. Food and Drug Administration 2008a) or other appropriate regulatory postmarket surveillance system.

Q7.3 I am a pediatric hematologist serving on a DMC for an experimental treatment for pediatric epilepsy. I have been placed on this DMC due to expected hematologic AEs. I have chaired several DMCs for other sponsors for treatments in pediatric anemia. The Chair of this DMC is a pediatric epileptologist. I have noticed that he has done quite a bit of work for this sponsor over the years and is always having small talk with sponsor representatives about other sponsor personnel that he knows before our open session begins. The other MD members of the DMC are all pediatric epileptologists and have known one another for many years. I am the new kid on the block. We are masked to treatment but during our closed session, he often plays down the importance of SAEs that we feel might be on the experimental arm or he attributes them to the active control. The other pediatric neurologists generally agree with him instantaneously. I have asked them to look closer at some of these SAEs but they are not hematological in nature so they feel that they know more about this than I do. We seem to be in a decision-making deadlock. What can I do about this?

A First, you and the biostatistician member of your DMC should remind the other members that you are free to comment on any safety issue that you think is important regardless of board certification. Ask the other members why they think the SAEs are due to the active control. Try to show any logical failures in their analysis if you can. Consult the literature and the active control package insert to learn of the SAEs expected. You can also consult with a pediatric epileptologist at your institution to see what he/she thinks of these SAEs and the active control. Of course, you cannot tell this person why you are asking but that should not be necessary. You can ask to be unmasked to the treatment assignments of just the patients that have the SAEs of your concern. Typically, the whole DMC should be unmasked. If they refuse at least you can be unmasked. If the SAEs are occurring more frequently on the experimental arm these steps should bring them out.

Q7.4 I am a sponsor representative working with a DMC in infectious disease. Our DMC has asked the DAC to prepare several ad hoc safety tables to address what they describe as an important concern. I approved the generation of these tables but three weeks have passed since the tables were completed and the DMC members can't agree on a date for their teleconference to go over the reports. We at the sponsor are concerned that patients are at risk and rumors are flying around the office which means that this information might have also reached the financial community. Part of the problem may be that because so many countries are represented in this trial that we have six physicians on the committee each representing a country being served.

A I would not recommend having fewer members on your DMC just because of problems in having ad hoc meetings. It is probably important to have six physician members but you must have six committed members, who are contactable wherever in the world they may be at the time an issue arises. However, the easiest way to address this problem might be to schedule a teleconference day before you approve the extra work for the DAC. The DAC must first tell you how much time they need to prepare the requested tables, listings, graphs, and so on. Once you have a commitment from all members to meet shortly after delivery you can approve the work order.

Q7.5 I am Chair of a DMC working on a cardiovascular indication. We have asked the DAC for several ad hoc reports to aid in the interpretation of safety concerns. The DAC tells us that they need several weeks for each table because of the need for validation of the software and cleaning of the data. We don't feel that we can take that much time given that patients are at risk. Can we overrule the need for validation and data quality control?

A You would not want to eliminate all software validation and data cleaning prior to generating the tables you need. You would not want to make decisions based on faulty data. In Table 3.1, we indicated that the extent of software validation and data quality control prior to data review was something to be entered into the DMC Charter before the trial begins. If the DAC has SOPs calling for certain validation procedures, it may be impossible to modify them. If they do not have SOPs for software validation for DMC operations, they should not have been selected as a DAC in the first place. The best procedure is to discuss a reasonable validation approach that gives the quality the DMC needs for its deliberations in the time frame that seems appropriate. If SOPs are being violated, a note can be written to the file detailing the reason for departure and the procedures that were followed.

Q7.6 I am an ophthalmologist serving on a DMC for an infectious disease of the eye. The other members are a retinologist who is serving as Chair, an internist, and a biostatistician. We have seen evidence of a very serious adverse event six weeks ago and I feel we should have told the sponsor to stop the trial now. The other members are asking for more information on the SAE reports, reading the literature including papers on animal studies that I do not feel them qualified to evaluate. Meanwhile patients are at risk. I am the only member of this DMC who treats patients of this type every day. I am growing frustrated at the amount of time the others have taken to investigate things that I know are irrelevant. Should I just contact the sponsor myself?

A Committee work has never been the most efficient way of doing business but you should not undervalue what the other members are doing just because it takes time. They may have a different but, nevertheless, important perspective. If the trial were to stop now, it will be difficult to start it again should your fellow committee members come up with information that might explain the SAEs and lead to recommendations for preventing these events. On the other hand, there may be people more qualified and more resources within the sponsor to deal with this issue. You ought to work with your fellow DMC members to establish a deadline for their research and then the DMC should brief the pharamacovigilence unit at the sponsor. The members of this group can be unmasked and can look into this matter without informing the study team of what is going on until a trial decision is needed. Also, the DMC does not have to tell this group that the trial should stop but merely that the sponsor gives the DMC reason why the trial should continue. You will find that the pharmacovigilence group has experience in dealing with these issues and should know how to proceed.

Q7.7 I am a cardiologist from Denmark serving as Chair of a DMC for a cardiovascular drug. The trial is being conducted in Europe. The sponsor is collecting the cost and quality of life data during this confirmatory trial in order to present to the U.K. NICE organization and the German IQWiG. The problem is that the sponsor is asking us to advise them on the quality and treatment differences of the cost and quality of life data along with the safety data. The cost and quality of life data take up so much of our time that I feel that we don't devote enough time to the safety data which we thought was our highest priority. In addition, the North American members of our DMC are not helping with the cost and quality of life data effort. They consider the data to be inadequate to answer any questions on cost-effectiveness. How can I get my committee back on track?

A You have encountered some of the problems of intercontinental differences in the drug approval process. Some European countries have the additional step of cost-effectiveness and North Americans are not used to cost-effectiveness being measured in the manner you describe. I do feel that safety should be a priority and I am sure that sponsor would agree. The sponsor should have made the cost-effectiveness responsibilities clear at the outset. At this point, you, as Chair, should discuss with the sponsor representative the possibility of their assembling another committee to review the cost and quality of life data. A one-person committee consisting of a knowledgeable consultant might be adequate for this purpose. If so, this individual could be added to the DMC to do this review while the rest of you work on safety.

Q7.8 I am serving as Chair of a DMC for colorectal cancer. Since our last meeting, the predetermined boundary for indication of futility was reached so that the DAC presented a very minimal safety analysis under the assumption that we would terminate the trial due to futility. Under what authority can they do that?

A This was bad practice on the part of the DAC. If the DAC did not receive instructions from the DMC regarding a revised analysis, they should provide the analysis that has been prespecified. Also, regardless of efficacy boundaries being crossed, there are still safety concerns to be discussed. If the trial is to be terminated, the DMC must consider continual treatment of patients in the experimental group and, despite futility, whether or not to recommend crossover to patients in the control group. The safety tables you prespecified would be an important resource for those recommendations. You must demand that the usual tables be sent to the DMC as soon as possible.

Q7.9 I am a neurologist serving on a DMC for a Parkinson's disease clinical trial. At our last meeting, we past the futility boundary but our Chair wanted to overrule the boundary because she felt that the experimental drug had a favorable safety profile and the trial would still serve as a noninferiority trial. Our biostatistical member felt this was OK. This did not sound right to me so I asked a statistical colleague at my institution who consults often with pharmaceutical firms and he said that arbitrary unplanned switching from superiority to noninferiority could not be done. For confidentiality reasons, I did not reveal the reason for my question to this colleague. I could call this to the attention of our biostatistical member but I could not argue the matter with her and, due to confidentiality, I cannot put her in touch with my academic colleague. Where do I go from here?

A There are a number of issues here. First, it is not clear that your DMC has the right to overrule a futility boundary and proceed with a plan B. Your committee's task is to inform the sponsor of the futility boundary being reached. You can recommend continuation because of the favorable safety profile but surely someone on the sponsor side would know, as your academic colleague correctly stated, switching from superiority to noninferiority can be done only by an approved adaptive design and with a preapproved indifference margin. The sponsor of your trial would be better served to terminate this superiority trial that your DMC is working on and design a separate noninferiority trial if that makes clinical and market sense to them. Your DMC's biostatistical member appears to be uninformed about certain statistical/regulatory technical details common to the pharmaceutical industry. This is not uncommon when academic biostatisticians with little previous connection to the pharmaceutical industry are placed on DMCs. After your trial is terminated, you and your academic colleague should inform her. This is all part of the training needed for the success of future DMCs.

Q7.10 I am Chair of a DMC working on a treatment for bladder cancer. The protocol calls for an interim nonbinding futility analysis with progression-free survival as the endpoint. The sponsor representative keeps changing the date of our face-to-face meeting because events are occurring at a slower rate than expected. It is always hard for us to all agree on a date for a meeting and it is annoying to have all these changes. Whenever I tell the sponsor representative that is difficult for the committee she just replies, "I'm sorry this analysis is driven by the number of events." What should I tell her the next time she changes a date?

A The news that progressions and/or deaths are occurring at a slow rate is good for the patients and their families and should be a nonissue between your DMC and sponsor. The problem of overestimating event occurrence is common so that most DMCs do not try to predict the precise date that the required number of events will occur and then schedule the meeting close to that date. Instead, they schedule the meeting several months after the predicted date to ensure that the number of events will be achieved. The criteria for this nonbinding futility analysis of progression-free survival will likely be calculated using the Lan–DeMets method. This method adjusts the criteria for the information time actually used. So, if your meeting does not take place at information time = 0.50 but rather 0.60 the correct criteria will be used. Tell your sponsor representative to relax, especially since this is a nonbinding futility analysis.

Q7.11 I am a physician member of a DMC for advanced breast cancer. We just completed a nonbinding futility analysis and did not cross the boundary. I have told my fellow members that we should terminate anyway because judging by the efficacy and safety we have seen and the cost of drugs in this class, the treatment will not be cost-effective. My fellow members think we should just follow the protocol and indicate that the boundary for termination has not been reached. Am I off base here?

A Cost-effectiveness of cancer treatments is certainly a timely topic. However, this is not a responsibility of the DMC, sponsor, or, in the United States, even the FDA. Moreover, there are no accepted criteria for cost-effectiveness. I hope you do not feel that your fellow DMC members are dismissive of your concerns. Perhaps, you can suggest an informal discussion on cost-effectiveness with the sponsor when the trial concludes.

Q7.12 I am the biostatistical member of a DMC for a drug for congestive heart failure. There was a planned interim analysis for efficacy and we saw the survival curves right on top of one another. We were also not enamored with the safety profile of this drug. We concluded that this trial should stop and communicated this to the sponsor team. About 3 days later, I got a call from an executive at the sponsor asking if we had computed conditional power. I was not comfortable talking to this person especially since I was not the DMC Chair. I told the executive to call the DMC Chair. We did not compute conditional power. It was not in the protocol. Should we have done that?

A The first problem is the executive had no right to call you and you were right to refer him to the Chair. It would be ideal if a DMC could ask for a conditional power calculation at any time even when not planned but, unfortunately, this is not commonly done. If you saw the survival curves on top of one another, then, under most drift assumptions, you would be calculating a small conditional power so I wouldn't worry about the lack of this calculation. Actually this matter could have been worse for the sponsor. Suppose you indicated that the trial should continue. At the final analysis, the sponsor sees that the survival curves were indistinguishable at the time of interim analysis as well as at final analysis. Would this executive now be calling you to ask "why in heaven's name did you not recommend termination at the interim?"

Q7.13 I am Chair of a DMC working on a drug for Parkinson's disease. A safety issue emerged and we asked the sponsor to supply a consulting group to the DMC to work on a meta-analysis of other trials of similar drugs to see how this drug compared for this SAE type. The sponsor refused at interim analysis when we did not want to specify what the specific SAE was for fear of unmasking but the sponsor also refused our request at the end of the trial after the protocol team was unmasked. We were let down about this. Do other DMCs succeed in having meta-analyses prepared?

A The use of meta-analysis for safety assessment is a new field. Conducting a meta-analysis is both an art and science and is not something to be rushed according to the aggressive timeline of a drug development program. Your request at interim probably confused the sponsor—what adverse event were you talking about? Was it a Tier 1 event? Who to contact to do such an analysis? How much would it cost? Can it be kept confidential? At the end of the trial is when the DMC has least clout. DMC responsibilities are now over. The sponsor at this point has enough work on their hands in dealing with investigators and regulators. If the drug were deemed approvable, the sponsor would probably feel that the meta-analysis might raise more questions than it answers and it could affect the drug label. Your request was a good one but, perhaps, about 5 years ahead of its time. Down the line, we should be able to rely on public databases to get a handle on your SAE of concern. Also, in Chapter 1, we described the safety assessment committee (SAC) that the FDA has recently recommended. Our current understanding of the broader scope of this committee would suggest that the SAC might be better prepared and better funded to request the meta-analysis.

Q7.14 I am the biostatistical member of a DMC working on a renal cancer drug. The active control can be called Treatment A and the experimental treatment can be called Treatment B. The trial randomized patients to Treatment A versus Treatments A + B. There was no planned interim analysis but we have seen a higher death rate in the A + B group than in the A group. The difference was statistically significant at the 0.03 significance level by my own analysis. The deaths were due to the disease and not toxicity. We were baffled by this observation. My physician colleagues reasoned that the experimental treatment might be interfering in some way with the known efficacy of the active control. We asked to speak to someone outside the sponsor's protocol team so as not to unmask and, ultimately, the senior biostatistician from the sponsor called me. He asked what I was worried about. This was a new trial. In time things will surely even out. Our request for a nonbinding futility conditional power analysis was denied. At the next analysis, the trend was the same but not quite statistically significant as before. We again asked for a conditional power calculation and the sponsor said that this was not called for in the protocol. What boundaries would we use? This is unchartered territory. Finally, a conditional power was calculated and we recommended termination on the basis of this analysis. Did this have to drag on so long?

A All this comes down to the ability of the DMC to request a conditional power analysis even if it is not already included in a planned interim analysis. Your analysis found statistical significance in the wrong tail. You were reasoning that if the home team in baseball is ahead 14-0 in the second inning, the end result of this game might not be a shutout but it is unlikely that the visiting team will win. The sponsor wanted to protect their drug and did not want the negative publicity of a trial ending so soon. The DMC's job was to protect patient safety. Yes, the conditional power analysis should have come immediately after your first calculation. However, the sponsor didn't know as much about the data as you did and had no rationale at hand for how the experimental treatment could interfere with the efficacy of the active control. This often results in a stalemate.

Q7.15 I was Chair of a recently completed clinical trial of a drug for a life-threatening disease. The primary endpoint was treatment failure defined as progression or death within 60 days of treatment start. The total sample size was 90 patients on each of the experimental treatment arm and placebo arm. Two futility analyses were planned at information times 0.33 and 0.67. The futility analysis was never specified as binding or nonbinding. At the first futility analysis, there were more deaths in the experimental arm than placebo but the same number of progressions. At this point, there were more patients with unfavorable prognostic factors on the experimental treatment. For these reasons, even though the futility boundary was crossed we decided to continue the trial. We crossed the futility boundary at the second interim analysis as well but the deaths in each group were even and the prognostic factors were beginning to balance. Owing to the life-threatening nature of this disease, we decided to continue because of the possibility that this drug could prolong life. At the final analysis, the prognostic factors were balanced; there were indeed more deaths in the placebo group but the experimental treatment failed in the primary endpoint because the percent of failures were about the same in each group. All the DMC members considered our decision making to be prudent but the sponsor is mad that we ignored the futility boundaries at the two interim analyses. They claim that all futility analyses are binding and we should have known that. The way we see it—fewer deaths in the experimental treatment and equal failures in the two groups—positive outcome. Why is there such a difference of opinion?

A I think this was a positive trial because there are many lessons to learn about the application of futility analysis. The first mistake was to use the term futility without the binding or nonbinding modifier. The protocol and DRP should have specified this. Scheduling an interim analysis at information time = 0.33 when there were only 30 patients in each group leads to your seeing the accidental imbalance in prognostic factors. The prognostic factors evened out at the end of trial as we would expect. The sponsor sees drug failure events progression and death to be equally weighted and the DMC weighted death higher. Perhaps, death should have been the primary endpoint. Unfortunately the formulas for futility boundaries do not adjust for prognostic factor imbalances. Even if they did, it is not clear how much of an adjustment you would have seen with such small sample sizes. Alas this trial was likely too small for even one futility analysis let alone two. You are correct; the result was not bad for the patients. As in most trials, lessons have been learned.

Q7.16 I am the biostatistical member of a solid tumor trial conducted by a Big Pharma sponsor. The drug is approved for other solid tumor indications and this trial is designed to assess the difference in overall survival between 1 and 2 years of treatment. Optimistically, the trial is planned for a total of 8 years. The patients randomized to the 1-year group receive a placebo for year 2. After year 2, all patients still in the trial are continued on standard of care. We have found no safety issues to date. An interim analysis of overall survival was performed for nonbinding futility after all patients completed 2 years on the trial. We found the two survival curves to be on top of one another and low conditional power for finding a statistically significant difference at the end of the trial regardless of drift assumption. Our Chair called the sponsor's vice president—oncology from our conference room. To our surprise, he said that we would continue the trial because nobody is being harmed. We were all upset by this decision. Shouldn't we be?

A Indeed you should be upset if not outraged. Your mentioning that this drug has already been approved for this indication and other solid tumors is a hint of what is going on. The VP wants to protect the brand. The sponsor does not want any negative information coming out about this product while it still has patent life. With a list of approved indications, there has probably been a string of successful trials and a report of a negative trial could change clinician opinion. I don't agree that nobody is being harmed. I wonder about the ethics if the patients are not to be debriefed at this point. With debriefing, the patients could opt to seek another treatment rather than wait for recurrence when it might be too late. Regardless, the patients are put through the rigor of making regular visits. True, this might be beneficial but they might opt to make regular visits to a primary care physician instead. In retrospect, this should have been a binding futility analysis.

Q7.17 I am the Chair of a DMC working on an Alzheimer's protocol for an Infant Pharma sponsor. The trial is being run by a large CRO. At the organizational meeting, our committee suggested the inclusion of an interim analysis for futility and the sponsor and regulators agreed. Our biostatistical member then asked the CRO to submit a mock table of conditional power to be used in this analysis. At our first data review meeting, a senior statistical advisor employed by the CRO joined the meeting by phone and said that conditional power is looked down upon by regulators because of its effect on Type I error (regulator's risk). He then described an unintelligible method for conducting the futility analysis that none of us, including our biostatistical member, understood. We let it pass but we know the date for the planned interim analysis is approaching. How do we get what we asked for?

A I had not heard of regulators not approving a conditional power analysis for futility. Moreover, this senior statistical advisor is wrong in implying that conditional power affects Type I error in any way. It affects Type II error (sponsor's risk) so this is not the regulators' concern. To proceed, I would just explain to the sponsor and CRO that your DMC feels the conditional power analysis is standard and that is what the DMC wants. Your biostatistical member might add that Type I error is not affected. Just explain this to the sponsor staff or the protocol staff at the CRO and let them pass on the word to the statistical advisor. I would suspect that you will not hear from him again.

8

Emerging Issues

PREVIEW We conclude this book with some emerging issues that are beginning to affect DMC operations today and will certainly do so in the future. We begin with adaptive designs and the challenges they place on DMC safety analysis. We then move on to two novel designs in oncology—umbrella trials and basket trials which have their own challenges. The SMART/DTS designs with their many branches, pragmatic trials, and biosimilar trials are all discussed. The use of patient-reported AE severity (PRO-CTCAE) and *in vitro* companion diagnostics are appearing more in trials. Both appear to be a consequence of the big push to precision medicine. The use of centralized risk-based monitoring replacing site monitoring implemented solely by CRA visits will give additional data quality responsibilities to the DMCs. Training of DMC members, the advent of internal safety review committees, and compensation of DMC members will be covered as well. Causal inference is entering the mainstream of clinical trial data analysis so we have included a brief introduction. There is no question that data fraud in clinical trials exists and the use of a Fraud Recovery Plan is described to salvage a clinical trial that has experienced fraud.

KEY WORDS: *adaptive design, umbrella design, basket design, SMART/DTS trials, pragmatic trials, PRO-CTCAE, biosimilar trials,* in vitro *companion diagnostics, centralized risk-based monitoring, causal inference, training of DMC members, internal safety review committees, Fraud Recovery Plan (FRP), 21st Century Cures Act*

8.1 Introduction

This chapter investigates recent trends in the pharmaceutical industry and how they might affect the operations of a DMC. The trends are divided into two broad categories—those related to changes in technology or company organization and those related to the maturity of DMCs as a clinical trial component.

8.2 Issues in New Clinical Trial Designs and Technologies

8.2.1 Adaptive Designs

The pharmaceutical industry has realized that there is a need to accelerate drug development because clinical trial design, analysis, and the regulatory process have not kept up with advances in technology. There are more compounds under investigation for more indications than has ever been the case previously. Many treatments will not make it to approval and sponsors want to eliminate these candidates as soon as possible in the development cycle. Those treatments that will be approved will have relatively short lifetimes due to competition and rapid technological advance. In the United States, FDA has acknowledged this need with their Critical Path Initiative (U.S. Food and Drug Administration 2004a). In this program, FDA is encouraging research in biomarkers, genetics, and statistical/clinical trial methodology to help in the needed acceleration. One of the principal statistical ideas for accelerating the clinical trial process is *adaptive designs*. Dragalin (2006) and Gallo and Krams (2006) have provided a good overview of the types of adaptive designs under consideration. An adaptive design is one that uses data accumulating during the clinical trial to change sample size, hypothesis, drop treatment groups, make a "seamless" transition from a phase II to a phase III trial, and so on, while preserving statistical properties such as Type I and Type II error. Obviously, drug development efficiency is gained in adapting a trial rather than beginning an additional trial using information from the previous trial. Discussion of the pros and cons of these proposed methods is beyond the scope of this book. However, Herson (2008) has discussed the effects of various types of adaptive designs on DMCs involved principally in safety monitoring. Gallo (2006) has offered some ideas for alterations in trial monitoring that might be necessary for adaptive designs.

The problem arises because adaptation is based on efficacy alone and the DMC is involved in periodic safety assessments independent of efficacy. To avoid unmasking and bias, the sponsor is unaware of adaptive changes being made. The challenge is what to do if safety concerns are in conflict with adaptive changes. Some examples follow.

8.2.1.1 Dropping a Dose or Treatment Group

Suppose a clinical trial with three experimental treatments or doses of the same treatment are being compared to a control group in an adaptive design trial that permits dropping an experimental group on the basis of efficacy. Clearly if the DMC is given word that a group is being dropped, they immediately know that this group was not the control group. However, we have already stated that there is no major problem in the DMC being unmasked to treatment. The problem occurs if the DMC has developed safety concerns about the groups that will remain in the trial but was comfortable with the developing safety profile of the treatment group being dropped. Upon being informed by the DAC biostatistician that the conditions for dropping this "safety-friendly" group have been met, the DMC might suddenly be discussing terminating the entire trial rather than continue with treatments that may demonstrate efficacy but do not have a favorable safety profile. This being an interim analysis, it may be too early for the DMC to look at efficacy data and evaluate risk versus benefit for the remaining groups. However, they must be careful in discussing a decision with the sponsor because the information divulged can introduce bias if the trial is to continue. The best solution would be for the DMC to begin a dialog with the sponsor about terminating the trial and not make a recommendation until sufficient discussion has taken place. This discussion should take place with sponsor staff not directly involved in the trial and only limited information about treatment performance should be given. A discussion with noninvolved sponsor staff might be possible for Big or Middle Pharma but not for Infant Pharma where everybody in the company has the potential of an emotional tie with the outcome of the trial. In these cases, CRO staff or the staff of a Big Pharma corporate partner may be able to participate in this dialog.

8.2.1.2 Adaptive Assignment to a Treatment Group

Under this scheme, the random allocation to treatment groups changes dynamically according to accumulating efficacy data with the treatments showing more efficacy potential being allocated to more patients. Here, the DMC will be very aware of efficacy because the safety tables they review will have more patients on the more favorable arms. Concerns may arise if these so-called favorable arms are also considered most toxic. The imbalance created by adaptive assignment may not permit adequate comparison of treatment groups for risk versus benefit. One solution would be for the DMC to recommend suspension of allocation change when imbalance becomes too large. Allocation can be changed again after the safety profile is considered better understood by the DMC.

For the remaining adaptive design sections, let's assume that there are only two treatment groups—experimental and control.

8.2.1.3 Changing Objectives: Superiority to Noninferiority

Much has been written about noninferiority trials and the statistical methodology involved (D'Agostino, Massaro, and Sullivan 2003). In the noninferiority trial, the objective is to show that the experimental treatment is at least not much worse in efficacy than an already-approved drug for this indication (active control). Presumably there is some benefit to the experimental treatment in terms of safety, convenience, cost, and so on. In a superiority trial in oncology, DMC physicians might be willing to accept grade 3–4 nausea and vomiting hoping that an improvement in overall survival will be demonstrated at the end of the trial. With a switch in objectives to noninferiority, the DMC will be told that the sponsor does not expect to demonstrate efficacy superiority against the active control. The physician DMC member mindset will often change at this point. Now, grade 3–4 nausea and vomiting in one arm (and known not to exist in the active control arm) becomes a reason to deem these treatments as not equivalent regardless of efficacy data. Some physician members will claim that inferiority of the experimental treatment has been demonstrated (not superior in efficacy, more toxic than control) and, hence, there is no reason to continue the trial. This situation would be less likely to happen if an adaptive change objectives design was not being used because in those cases, the sponsor would usually have sufficient evidence of a favorable safety profile before beginning the trial. In an adaptive design, the safety profile is usually not that well known at the time the trial begins and, hence, this kind of situation can occur occasionally. It is not clear what the communication between the DMC and sponsor should be in this case. The DMC may not have a safety *concern* but more of an observation of a safety *differential* between treatments which would deem the experimental treatment inferior to the active control. A DMC recommendation of trial termination appears appropriate in this case.

8.2.1.4 Seamless Transition: Phase II to Phase III

Seamless transition can take place where efficacy data support proceeding from phase II to phase III. The patients already enrolled in the phase II trial become part of the phase III trial and the sample size is increased to pivotal trial levels. At the time of transition, the DMC may have already developed safety concerns and believe that it is inappropriate to increase sample size. This situation appears simpler than those cited above and is one that occurs in the practice of sample size reestimation (Chuang-Stein, Anderson, Gallo et al. 2006). In most protocols that allow for sample size reestimation through an interim analysis, it is understood that sample size increase can only take place if the sponsor has no safety concerns that would preclude increasing sample size. Thus, seamless transition can easily be absorbed by DMC operations under sample size reestimation.

8.2.1.5 Change in Effect Size of Interest

A popular method of *sample size reestimation* is the *CHW method* of Cui, Hung, and Wang (1999). This scheme uses a conditional power calculation at a planned interim analysis to compute the sample size necessary to deliver the required power for the *observed* effect size. An odds ratio of 2.0 in favor of the experimental treatment may have been agreed upon at the start of the trial but an odds ratio of 1.4 is observed at the interim analysis. An increase in sample size at this point is indicative of a change to a smaller effect size than that agreed upon as clinically significant at the beginning of the trial. The sponsor realizes that, if this smaller effect size is found statistically significant at the end of the trial, they will have to convince regulatory authorities that the revised effect size is of clinical significance. However, DMC members will be aware of the change in effect size at the interim analysis. It has already been mentioned that risk versus benefit is a difficult task during or even at the conclusion of a single pivotal trial. It is even more difficult when the benefit (effect size of interest) is a moving target. Some DMC members may feel that the emerging safety profile cannot be justified with the smaller effect size. This would be the reason to terminate the trial. Under these circumstances, the DMC may recommend to the sponsor that safety considerations dictate that the effect size of interest not be changed. There would not be a reason to indicate what the safety concerns are at this point. The sponsor may choose to terminate the trial due to the futility of finding the original effect size statistically significant at the end of the trial.

A summary of DMC communications and actions in adaptive designs is found in Table 8.1.

8.2.1.6 Further Thoughts on Adaptive Designs

It must be clear that adaptive clinical trial designs, other than sample size reestimation, are a new concept for pivotal trials. There are many details to be worked out to satisfy concerns of sponsors, investigators, and regulators. The discussion above was only intended to mention some issues that a DMC focusing on safety issues might face when adaptation based on efficacy is about to take place. Besides concern, when the experimental treatment's efficacy and safety characteristics appear to diverge, there is the problem of what is the proper DMC–sponsor communication about the concerns that does not introduce bias into trial operations. It probably makes sense for protocols to provide for a period of "white space" (period of time reserved for planning) whenever adaptation takes place. During this period, the DMC would be asked to comment on safety concerns before the adaptation could take place. The problem remains of what sponsor unit would receive this report. Later in this chapter, we will discuss the appearance of internal safety review committees which are beginning to appear in Big Pharma. These committees consist of physicians and biostatisticians employed by the company but not working on this trial. The rationale for this will be discussed below. For Big Pharma using the internal committee, the DMC could presumably report to this body. Such a unit would not exist in Infant Pharma and, for these sponsors, the DMC will have to issue a carefully worded statement. One alternative is for adaptive design trials not to be used at all until previous trials establish the safety profile. For sponsors of all sizes, physicians may be reluctant to become involved in DMCs for pivotal trials when the investigator brochure for the experimental drug is sparse on safety.

TABLE 8.1

Summary of DMC Issues and Actions in Trials with Efficacy-Based Adaptation

Efficacy-Based Adaptation Type[a]	Issue	Data Monitoring Committee Action
Drop dose or treatment group	The dose/treatment group being dropped might be the only one in the trial with an acceptable safety profile	Begin a dialog with sponsor representative on the need for trial termination
Adaptive assignment to treatment group	Random treatment allocation is favoring a treatment arm with an unfavorable safety profile	Either ask sponsor to change allocation to equal per treatment group until safety profile becomes clear, recommend elimination of unsafe treatment group, or trial termination
Changing objectives— superiority to noninferiority	Regardless of efficacy unfavorable safety profile in experimental group means treatments are not equivalent	Recommend trial termination
Seamless transition phase II to phase III	Sponsor is aware of this transition and will consult DMC for possible safety concern before proceeding to phase III	Recommend transition if no safety concern
Changing effect size of interest	DMC members may feel that the emerging safety profile of the experimental treatment cannot be justified by a decreased efficacy effect size of interest derived by a conditional power calculation at an interim analysis	Recommend that the effect size of interest remains as originally planned if that effect size can be justified by safety risk or terminate the trial

Source: Herson, J., *Drug Inf. J.*, 42, 297–301, 2008.
[a] Communicated to Data Monitoring Committee by Data Analysis Center staff.

Both the biostatistician member and the DAC biostatistician must believe in and be well versed in adaptive methods and be able to explain them to the physician members. The physician members must also be comfortable with the adaptive approach before agreeing to serve on the DMC. Before any data review meeting where adaptation is a possibility, the two biostatisticians must lead the physician members through a decision matrix of steps that will take place contingent on the data to be reviewed. The rationale for each branch of the matrix must be carefully explained. This is best done before members receive the data to be reviewed at the meeting. A conference call can be used for this purpose and timed to take place before data are sent to members.

8.2.2 Novel Designs in Oncology

The *umbrella design* and the basket design are attempts to speed up the drug discovery process in oncology.

The umbrella design is a master protocol for a single tumor type but several experimental drugs each targeted to a specific biomarker or genetic mutation are rotated in and out according to efficacy criteria. Hence, this is also an advance in precision (personalized) medicine. The design generally employs a common control group. This is a cooperative venture among several sponsors. Drugs are eliminated if they do not show efficacy to any biomarker type by frequentist criteria but are elevated to phase III trial status via a Bayesian predictive model. Examples of umbrella trials are ISPY-2, a neoadjuvant breast cancer trial (Barker, Sigman, Kelloff et al. 2009), ALCHEMIST for early-stage non-small-cell lung cancer (Gerber, Oxnard, and Govindan 2015), and Lung-MAP for advanced squamous cell lung cancer (Herbst, Gandara, Hirsch et al. 2015).

The challenge for DMCs with the umbrella design is that, being a master protocol, the trial never closes so there will have to be a rotation of DMC members preferably with interlocking terms. There will be limited safety information from some drugs that don't last on the protocol very long but DMCs will be very important in making recommendations on those drugs being elevated to phase III. Perhaps, one member of the DMC should follow that drug to chair the phase III DMC. DMCs will also advise when enrollment cohorts should expand or cease and decide when to release data and to which parties.

Closely related to the umbrella trial is the *basket trial*. This is also a precision medicine master protocol trial but this trial takes patients that have genetic mutations of interest regardless of tumor type. This protocol will have drugs on the shelf to use with patients of given mutations and, as in the umbrella trials, these drugs will be rotated in and out according to efficacy criteria. Examples of basket trials are NCI-MATCH (McNeill 2015) and the American Society of Clinical Oncology (ASCO) TAPUR study (clinicaltrials.gov 2016). The latter is a nonrandomized registry of experience with FDA-approved drugs with various mutation types. The DMC responsibilities with the basket trials are similar to those of the umbrella trials except that in the basket trials, the DMC will not necessarily have members with tumor-specific expertise. Since patients are enrolled by biomarker type, there may not be, for example, a renal cell tumor specialist on the panel. However, the direction of the basket trial is that tumor type does not matter as much as biomarker type.

8.2.3 Dynamic Treatment Strategies (DTS) and a Sequential Multiple Assignment Randomization Trial (SMART)

The *SMART/DTS trial designs* have been described by Lavori and Dawson (2014). Patients are randomized to two treatments at the commencement of the trial but the protocol for these trials specifies various decision points where subsequent randomization is to be performed. For example, patients experiencing unacceptable toxicity might be randomized between a lower dose for this drug or a different drug. Patients who meet a definition of response might now be randomized between two maintenance regiments. Those patients whose disease progresses might now be randomized to either of two drugs but the choices would be different depending on what maintenance regimen the patient was on at the time of progression. Thus, the trial develops into a decision tree diagram with the number of patients who will fall into each branch unknown at the beginning of the trial. Habermann, Weller, Morrison et al. (2006) conducted a fairly simple trial of this type in B-cell lymphoma.

The DTS/SMART trial is considered an improvement over the intent-to-treat interpretation where patients are randomized to a policy of beginning treatment with drug A or drug B and analysis compares these two drugs regardless of how clinicians might change treatment regimen as events occur over time. While the intent-to-treat principle is scientifically correct, there is always a question of its generalizability because in practice response to events might be handled differently by different clinicians. In the DTS/SMART scheme, there is randomization at every event/decision point which would be expected to make for a more useful comparison. The final data from a DTS/SMART design can be analyzed to define an optimal treatment regimen but, presumably, this branch would have to be compared with other contenders in a traditional confirmatory trial.

DMCs working on a DTS/SMART trial would face several challenges and those challenges would multiply depending on the number of branches that develop. The DMC might find fewer cases of toxicity than in a traditional trial if patients are randomized to alternate regimens at the time of toxicity. Ultimately they will have to look at the branches where most patients fell and try to trace what decision points along the way might have minimized or exacerbated the adverse events. Fortunately most DTS/SMART designs are being conducted in the postmarket so few surprises are expected in the area of safety.

8.2.4 Pragmatic Trials and Patient-Reported Outcomes of Safety

The definition of pragmatic clinical trials has varied over the years but more recently this term has been applied to trials that have the objective to inform decisions on medical interventions rather than an explanatory trial that would have the objective of gaining a better understanding of how or why an intervention works (Califf and Sugarman 2015). The pragmatic trial seeks to enroll patient populations relevant to informing the decision makers (clinicians, health insurers, patients, etc.) and allows interventions loosely defined and applied by clinicians in real-world settings. The emergence of electronic medical records at all levels of clinical practice should allow the enrollment of clinicians as investigators and their patients as clinical trial subjects (Califf, Filerman, Murray et al. 2012).

PAC-Man is an example of a pragmatic clinical trial (Harvey, Harrison, Singer et al. 2005). The pulmonary artery catheter (PAC) is a widely used hemodynamic monitoring device in the management of critically ill patients though doubts exist about its safety. The objective was to do a randomized trial in a real-world setting to see whether hospital mortality is reduced in critically ill patients when they are managed by a PAC. A total of 1041 patients were randomized to management with and without PACs. No specific instructions were given to the clinics as to patient management with or without the PAC. The conclusion was that there was no difference in hospital mortality between PAC and non-PAC management. The authors make it clear that PAC-Man was an effectiveness trial and that an efficacy trial with a rigid protocol for use might provide different results but the point is that PAC-Man showed its audience of clinicians, health insurers, and patients that there is no risk–benefit advantage in the real-world setting.

Ellenberg, Culbertson, Gillen et al. (2015) describe the use of data monitoring committees for pragmatic trials. They indicate that DMCs will have to be involved in pragmatic trials because of their potential impact on clinical practice. Surely there is a need to monitor safety, patient eligibility, and patient follow-up but it is not clear that patient adherence with the intervention or the clinician's patient management need to be monitored because to do so would steer the trial away from pragmatic and move toward an efficacy trial. It will be important that DMC members understand the difference between the pragmatic and explanatory (efficacy) trials and are grounded in the real world rather than the academic setting.

There has long been a feeling that investigator description and grading of adverse events does not reflect the true impact of the event on the patient. While the classification may be clinically correct, it does not carry information on the emotional toll or the interference with daily activities that only the patient can describe. As a result in oncology trials, where so many adverse events are observed, the U.S. National Cancer Institute has been working with investigators in developing a patient-reported outcomes version of the CTCAE (Common Terminology Criteria for Adverse Events). It is known as PRO-CTCAE (U.S. National Cancer Institute 2013, 2016). The PRO-CTCAE measurement system is an online real-time system for patients to report adverse events as they occur. A library of symptomatic adverse events has been created and sponsors would, presumably, only select the AESIs or other types of adverse events that may not be reliably reported by investigators for PRO-CTCAE reporting. Patients are asked to report symptom occurrence and frequency. A grading system from 1 to 5 is used to bring severity and interference with body function and daily routine. Dueck, Mendoza, Mitchell et al. (2015) have reported on the validity and reliability of the PRO-CTCAE with positive results.

DMCs should expect to receive direct patient reporting of adverse events in clinical trials in the future. The DMC must make sure that the sponsor takes the patient reporting as seriously as investigator reporting and that patient reporting has at least equal weight with investigator reporting in their decision making.

8.3 Biosimilar Designs

While chemical-based drugs can be approved for generic competition by a relatively straightforward pharmacokinetic regulatory pathway this is not the case for biologics. The FDA has created a *biosimilar* pathway for follow-on biologics. The regulatory details and design and analysis insights for biosimilar programs are described by Chow (2014). Not all biosimilars will have to undergo clinical trials but those that do will be in a randomized bioequivalence design comparing the branded product with the experimental biosimilar. In biosimilar trials, there will be much interest in the efficacy endpoint. DMCs will also have to keep a close eye on safety to see that the expected adverse events are occurring with equal frequency in each group and be quick to inform the sponsor if the experimental arm has a disproportionate frequency of the expected AEs and/or if new types of AEs are observed. In a biosimilar trial for the breast cancer biologic trastuzumab, for example, the protocol may allow each site to use a different taxane on each arm. The DMC members will have to be knowledgeable of differential AEs between the taxanes as well and keep track of which sites are using paclitaxel and which are using docetaxel. A vigil on patient and clinician compliance with protocol will also be important.

8.4 *In Vitro* Companion Diagnostic Devices

As we enter the era of precision medicine, eligibility for clinical trials is often based on patients having a certain biomarker. Determining eligibility requires that a patient be screened using an *in vitro* companion diagnostic device. The protocol for these trials must describe the specific *companion diagnostic device* to be used and this device must also go through regulatory approval (U.S. Food and Drug Administration 2014). The field of precision medicine is new and, hence, the *in vitro* companion diagnostics specified in protocols are often going through the regulatory process at the time that the trial using the biomarker is in progress. This means that some patients may be screened using an assay and others with the companion diagnostic after approval and a bridging study might be needed.

As part of its regular vigil over patient accrual, the DMC will have to watch the percent of patients who pass the eligibility screening and, if this percent is lower than expected, ask the sponsor for a revised schedule for a planned interim analysis, trial completion date, and so on. The DMC will also advise on the need to enroll new sites, increase recruitment procedures for existing sites with poor enrollment, and so on. The DMC must monitor the approval process of the companion diagnostic and decide if the sensitivity, specificity, and diagnostic accuracy of the diagnostic is satisfactory for trial integrity.

Table 8.2 summarizes the DMC issues for the emerging clinical trial designs.

TABLE 8.2

Summary of DMC Issues for Emerging Clinical Trial Designs

Design	Description	DMC Issues
Umbrella	Single tumor type, many drugs rotated in and out, and related to biomarkers or genetic mutations.	Trial never closes, DMC members must rotate, and some drugs may be elevated to their own phase III trial with limited safety information.
Basket	Patients are classified by genetic mutation rather than by tumor type. Drugs are rotated in and out according to the biomarkers they target.	Same issues as umbrella but in the basket the DMC won't necessarily have members with expertise in the range of tumor types.
Dynamic treatment strategies (DTS)/ sequential multiple assignment randomization trials (SMART)	As events such as SAE or progression occur, the clinician does not make a decision of what to do, the protocol randomizes patients to a specific decision.	DMC members will have to trace back branches to ascertain what may have lead up to the adverse events. However, at least the branches will be standardized and not up to clinician discretion.
Pragmatic trials	Performed in real-world settings, minimal inclusion criteria, and administration of the treatment is left up to the clinician.	DMC members might get confused with the real world vs. academic setting and try to steer the trial away from pragmatic and toward detailed protocol-driven treatments.
Patient-reported outcomes (PRO-CTCAE)	Patients grade their adverse events on a scale from 1 to 5 according to severity and interference with body function and daily routine.	DMC members must be on board with PROs and must make sure that the sponsor gives them equal weight with investigator grading.
Biosimilar designs	Bioequivalence designs for biologics.	Sponsor may be concentrating on efficacy outcomes but DMC must watch both arms to see that expected AEs are occurring with equal frequency in each group.
In vitro companion diagnostic devices	Diagnostics that screen patients for biomarkers that are eligibility criteria for the trial.	DMCs must monitor percent of patients passing screening and, if the passing rate is too low suggest ways of increasing enrollment. DMCs must review diagnostic accuracy of the companion diagnostic to make sure it meets standards.

8.5 Real-Time SAE Reporting Using the Internet

Many sponsors are using Internet-based collaboration software for DMC support. This software allows DMC members to view various documents throughout the trial. In some clinical trials, individual SAE reports reach DMC members via an e-mail request to go to an Internet website to view the report. This e-mail is generated as soon as the SAE arrives at the sponsor. This type of real-time reporting is useful after a DMC has developed a safety concern such as early deaths, cardiovascular disease, and so on, and decides to monitor the situation closely before making a final decision. However, for all SAE reports to be reported in this way has the potential effect of creating attitudes among DMC members before reviewing cohort data. These attitudes could result in premature unmasking if the DMC is to remain masked or becoming overly conscious of a certain SAE type and ignoring others. A compromise might be for the real-time SAE reports to go only to the DMC Chair or a mutually agreed-upon other member. The Chair would decide if there is reason for an ad hoc meeting or for additional data review tables for the next DMC meeting that might clarify the situation.

All the new and proposed wearable technologies such as censors embedded in clothing, toilets and elsewhere in the home, high-tech wristwatches, nanoparticles in the drugs, and so on, will be connected to the Internet. These technologies will be able to send information and possible adverse events to sponsors and regulators in real time. The technologies will be able to determine patients overdosing, under dosing, taking drugs not permitted by the protocol, and so on. Eventually, this type of information will come to the DMC. The members will have to specify if they want to be bombarded with a continuous flow of data or they would prefer to have the data integrated with the periodic reports they receive at DMC meetings. In the coming years, it is likely that sponsors will provide DMC members with statistical/graphics software with which they can manipulate data arriving from case report forms together with data coming from these new technologies and possibly even do analyses from databases containing data from outside the trial as described in Chapter 7. While this will give the DMC members considerable freedom but the possibility of each member reaching a different conclusion, using improper statistical methods, making comparisons that are not valid is considerable. The availability of the data might create an overzealous attempt to find harm in a drug. The incorporation of these technologies into the safety monitoring process will take time. Topol (2012) and Herson (2015b) provide a good overview of the new medical technologies and their implications.

8.6 Centralized Risk-Based Monitoring

For many decades, data quality and protocol adherence was monitored at each site by clinical research associates (CRAs) dispatched by the sponsor or the CRO. As the number of sites expanded and clinical trials began being conducted on a global basis, this type of monitoring was not scalable. In addition, because the monitoring was not focused, the site monitoring was not effective in creating data of the highest quality. Realizing that it was now possible to use statistical methods to find sites in need of improvement in data quality, the FDA issued a guidance indicating that centralized risk-based monitoring based on statistical and graphical methods could replace routine site monitoring (U.S. Food and Drug Administration 2013). Shortly thereafter, sophisticated statistical software began to appear for use in risk-based monitoring. Methodology and software are described by Venet, Doffagne, Burzykowski et al. (2012), Kirkwood, Cox, and Hackshaw (2013), and Timmermans, Venet, and Burzykowski (2016). The SAMIT trial, a phase III trial in gastric cancer used centralized statistical monitoring exclusively (Tsuburaya, Yoshida, Kobayashi et al. 2014). The specific methodology used in this trial is described by Timmermans, Doffague, Venet et al. (2016).

Centralized risk-based monitoring does not completely replace the CRA site monitoring. Rather, it directs fewer CRAs on fewer visits to address important issues.

As a result of this technology, DMC members will be able to receive data quality and protocol adherence metrics for each site on the trial. Updated metrics can be provided at each data review meeting. This will enable DMC members to advise sponsors on sites needing improvement and specify corrective action. This will bring DMCs more into the realm of sponsor operations and should result in more efficient clinical trials. The use of centralized statistical monitoring can also detect patterns of data that cannot be attributed to innocent errors but rather to fraud. The role of sponsors and DMCs in dealing with fraud detected in this manner will be discussed below.

8.7 Causal Inference

An exciting area of statistical research is the development of methods of causal inference (Rosenbaum and Rubin 1983; Frangakis and Rubin 2002). These methods use the statistical techniques of propensity scores and principal stratification to allow for adjustment of posttreatment variables that allow for conclusions of causation. One safety application that a DMC might encounter would be a post hoc analysis of safety based on variables measured during the trial. Suppose a DMC is monitoring a clinical trial for an oral pain medication and discovers a rate of cardiovascular disease in the experimental group much higher than that in the placebo group. It is also discovered that some patients overdosed the medication. Sponsor staff might perform a causal analysis of the effect of overdosing on the outcome of cardiovascular disease even though patients were not randomized on the basis of compliance with dose. This could lead to protracted discussions if the causal analysis revealed that it was overdosing and not the experimental treatment that caused the cardiovascular disease. Presumably there would still be evidence against the experimental treatment such as overdosing being caused by perceived lack of efficacy by the patient. In any case, the DMC biostatistician might not be selected on the basis of familiarity with causal inference methodology because, at the beginning of the trial, nobody thought such an analysis would be performed. This could be especially problematic if this analysis were done in response to a DMC observation of excess cardiovascular risk at an interim analysis rather than at the end of the trial. The resolution of this issue will depend on the specifics of the drug and the indication. However, if such an analysis were performed at the end of the trial, the DMC would, presumably, have no problem with the analysis appearing in a manuscript for the trial and the regulatory agency would have input into how this analysis might be presented in a package insert. If this analysis occurs at interim analysis, the DMC would have to take it into consideration in a decision on trial termination.

Brooks, Go, Singer et al. (2015) apply causal inference to an observational study on safety in order to analyze it as if it were a randomized clinical trial.

Their objective is to evaluate the safety of warfarin in prevention of stroke for patients with atrial fibrillation. The adverse event of interest is bleeding. While randomized clinical trials have supported the efficacy and safety of warfarin for this indication, clinicians are wary of this conclusion because the trial patients with comorbidities are not eligible for these trials and these are the real-world patients at risk. Using the ATRIA-1 Cohort from the Kaiser Permanente Northern California database, they estimate the causal effect of nonstroke death during the first 12 months of treatment. This is done by adjusting for the factors that would lead to warfarin prescription. Their analysis finds no evidence that warfarin reduces nonstroke death and, in fact may increase risk due to the associated bleeding events. This study also shows that we may see more observational studies analyzed as clinical trials using these methods and such analyses may come before DMCs in the future.

Gibbons and Amatya (2016) also present methods of causal analysis to drug safety data with examples of smoking cessation drugs and suicidal behavior and children/adolescent use of antidepressants and suicidal behavior with a particular emphasis on using causal methods to correct for confounders.

8.8 Unmasking Potential of Biomarkers

The discovery of biomarkers for patient response, and their use as surrogate endpoints in clinical trials, have the potential of increasing efficiency in clinical trials. However, recent clinical trials in oncology have shown that the epidermal growth factor drugs cetuximab (Lenz, Van Cutsem, Khambata-Ford et al. 2006) and erlotinib (Wacker, Nagrani, Weinberg et al. 2007) are associated with skin rashes and the severity of the rash is correlated with survival time. Thus, observation of an adverse event reveals information on efficacy. This is a problem for sponsor pharmacovigilence staffs. They are supposed to review adverse events but be masked to efficacy. There is no major problem of DMC members being aware of these data but they must be careful about discussing concerns about skin rashes with sponsor staff. The pharmacovigilence unit is a vital part of the safety monitoring process and they should not be shut out of safety data review. A possible solution is for one pharmacovigilence employee who does not work on oncology to receive all adverse event reports first and remove the skin rash reports. The remaining reports would be given to the oncology pharmacovigilence staff. If the skin rash reviewer sees a problem in volume or severity of skin rashes he/she can inform the DMC Chair. It is expected that more biomarkers related to efficacy in the form of adverse events will be discovered in the near future and there will be a need for further development of procedures of this type.

8.9 Issues Due to Maturing of DMC Processes and Evolution of the Pharmaceutical Industry

The use of DMCs in safety monitoring has become standard in most pharmaceutical industry confirmatory trials. As a result, questions other than appropriate content of the DMC Charter or number of members arise. We will examine some of these issues as well as some that arise from the evolution of the pharmaceutical industry.

8.9.1 Training of DMC Members

In the early days of DMCs in pharmaceutical industry clinical trials and as the DMC concept developed members received on-the-job training. At first, there were few people available to serve on DMCs that had the experience to train others and sponsors were putting together SOPs, which, initially, varied considerably from company to company. The guidance documents from regulatory agencies have helped in harmonization of procedures. The question that arises is whether or not on-the-job training is still the best preparation for DMC service or should formal training programs be organized. The latter would consist of Internet courses, apprenticeships, and certification. Of course, those who have served on DMCs would automatically be certified.

Training could take place through courses given online or at meetings of the Drug Information Association, Regulatory Affairs Professionals Association, Association of Clinical Research Professionals, British Institute of Regulatory Affairs, and so on. The written syllabus would consist of material presented in this book but role-playing and apprenticeship would also be part of an ideal program. Surely the emergences of massive online open courses (MOOCs) present an opportunity for training DMC members and sponsor staff. Organizations such as Coursera and edX could, presumably, partner with industry groups like the Drug Information Association, Clinical Trials Transformation Initiative, and so on, to create online courses as at least one step in the certification process. An online training program based on this book is currently available from statistics.com. Zuckerman, van de Schalie, and Cahill (2015) present their results of an exhaustive data-gathering program on the content for a DMC training program and have created modules for use at the National Institute of Allergic and Infectious Diseases.

The pros for a formal training program would be that it would allow younger professionals to serve on DMCs who might otherwise not be considered due to lack of experience. Diversity of DMC members would have many advantages over a smaller aging power elite of DMC members. An international registry of DMC professionals at varying certification status would help sponsors staff DMCs. As North American and European societies become more multicultural so are the patients who volunteer for clinical trials. It is important that this ethnic diversity be represented on DMCs.

The cons for such a program would include potential members not having the time or be willing to pay the expense for the training out of their own pocket. Apprenticeship training would require that sponsors pay the DMC members-in-training some stipend for meeting attendance and reimburse for travel expenses. Several people have proposed this to sponsors and been turned down.

If apprenticeship defined as having an extra person in the room is not feasible, perhaps, some use can be made in replacing members who find it necessary to resign from DMCs with potential trainees. Occasionally DMC members must resign due to change of employment, no longer being able to commit the time, illness, and so on. If such resignations occur late in the trial, adding a person at the trainee level would not require additional expense on the part of sponsors and the trainee would benefit from sitting in on a DMC that, by this time, has well-understood responsibilities and knowledge of the safety issues.

DMC training should also be provided to sponsor staff who will be working with DMCs but have no previous experience. Several experienced DMC members have had the experience of doing on-the-job training of sponsor staff who would otherwise not know how to conduct open meetings, what data review tables are required, coordinating data flow between sponsor, DAC and DMC, and so on. It should not be the responsibility of the DMC members to train sponsor staff. Sponsors can create internal programs to train their staff members and apprenticeships consisting of attendance at DMC meetings with more experienced sponsor staff. Other groups who might benefit from training in DMC operations would include persons wishing to perform DMC audits (see Section 8.9.3) and CROs that might want to serve as DACs.

If sponsors wanted to replace a resigning member with a trainee as described above, they would be encouraged to use those listed in the directory described above who have the desired educational and professional characteristics but no previous DMC experience.

8.9.2 Cost Control

In their deliberations, DMCs frequently see the need for ad hoc meetings and ad hoc tables and listings in order to better understand emerging safety issues. They may even ask to have an ad hoc consultant appointed such as a cardiologist or an immunologist/allergist for guidance in interpreting adverse events lying within their expertise. The DMC must be careful in making these requests because they do not want to unmask sponsor staff. As there is more experience with requests of this type, sponsors are asking should they be required to pay for this additional work without having input into the decision. All too often, sponsors have been getting bills for thousands of dollars for extra work only to find that the DMC ultimately decided there was no safety concern. At the end of the trial, sponsor staff are unmasked and, viewing the data, wonder why the ad hoc requests were made (see *DMCounselor* Q8.2 below).

Closely related to the cost control issue is ad hoc requests made to the DAC other than just generating additional tables with more granularity in a certain organ classification. For example, there may be requests for conditional power calculations, causal inference methods, or combining MedDRA preferred term codes across SOCs. Besides the cost of these activities, the requests may involve capabilities that the DAC staff does not have because the DAC was selected on the basis of different criteria. This is especially true when the DAC is based at a CRO working under contract with the sponsor. However, it can occur as well when the DAC is a separate unit within the sponsor.

One way of handling this would be for the DMC and the DAC to have a certain discretionary budget for ad hoc requests. This means that the DMC Chair will have to ask the DAC for the cost of the ad hoc requests and determine if the budget will be exceeded. If the budget is to be exceeded, or if consultants must be retained, the DMC will have to make carefully worded requests to the sponsor. The sponsor will have the right to veto the requests but there may be a middle ground such as reducing costs in other areas perhaps by eliminating routine tables that are no longer needed. If the sponsor vetoes, their representative should present the sponsor's rationale for the veto to the DMC. The rationale should not be merely that the request is too expensive. Often, the sponsor staff will have considerable information on mechanisms of action and pathways that may explain adverse events that DMC members deem important but do not have this deep knowledge of the drug.

8.9.3 DMC Audit

During the process of drug development, audits of investigator sites, CROs, sponsor records, manufacturing facilities, and clinical laboratories are common (International Conference on Harmonisation 1996). The audit process has recently included DMCs. The audits may be performed by the FDA or by the sponsor in anticipation of an FDA audit. Another pharmaceutical firm thinking of licensing the drug the DMC is monitoring might also want to make an audit. A DMC audit would consist of going over the charter and minutes of DMC meetings. The auditor would want to ascertain that the charter was followed, patient safety was under the stewardship of an independent DMC, there were no obvious conflicts of interest among DMC members, and there was no unmasking, accidental or otherwise, that could bias trial conduct. An important document in this audit would be the DMC minutes. These minutes would be prepared by the DMC secretary or the DAC biostatistician. There would be both open session and closed session minutes. In order for these minutes to be available for inspection at any time, there must be a record retention procedure in place. No records should be maintained in the home or office of a DMC member. The open session minutes can be stored by the sponsor clinical staff but the combination open–closed meeting minutes should be stored at the DAC or at some office of the sponsor separate from those involved in the trial such as a manufacturing or quality control office.

8.9.4 Internal Safety Review Committees and Still More Committees

The *internal safety review committee* (ISRC) is a fairly new phenomenon in Big Pharma. The ISRC is structured like a DMC with physician members and usually one biostatistician. All members are employees of the sponsor but work in other disease areas. The ISRC follows a charter similar to the DMCs as far as masking is concerned. The DMC meets only periodically and some Big Pharma sponsors feel there is a need to having an internal group meeting more frequently than a DMC can. The ISRC receives the same information as the DMC. The ISRC does not make unilateral decisions. They might hold ad hoc teleconferences with the DMC when important safety issues arise. The biostatistician member of the ISRC is usually the DAC biostatistician for the trial. The physician members of the ISRC might attend closed sessions of the DMC.

The use of an ISRC in a clinical trial brings many changes to the sponsor–DMC relationship and the data flow between sponsor, DAC, and DMC. Most importantly it raises the question of who is ultimately responsible for the stewardship of the trial. Having the ISRC as part of DMC discussions on safety might change the direction of decisions because, while some may question whether a DMC is truly independent of the sponsor, surely the ISRC is less independent. This is a new concept and, if an ISRC is to be involved in a trial, the DMC Charter should spell out the precise roles of each unit in detail. The DMC should make sure that the regulatory agencies involved are aware of the presence of the ISRC.

The ISRC should be distinguished from pharmacovigilence committees (sometimes called firewall or medical governance committees) mentioned earlier. These committees do not regularly review data on the trial as the ISRC does. They exist for consultation with the DMC when serious safety concerns arise which cannot be discussed with the sponsor staff because of unmasking potential.

Chapter 1 has already mentioned potential tensions when, in addition to a DMC, a steering committee is present in the trial. The importance of defining the responsibilities and limitations of each group before the start of the trial cannot be overemphasized. Chapters 1 and 7 also mention the recent FDA draft guidance (U.S. Food and Drug Administration 2015a) calling for the formation of a Safety Assessment Committee whose members would deal with safety issues on a particular trial but analyze them with broader scope.

It is likely that the day will come when we will see the emergence of meta data monitoring committees. Committees sponsored by industry and/or regulatory agencies would review safety data from a defined class of drugs both premarket and postmarket and make recommendations to regulators regarding safety policy.

The question "do we really need all of these committees?" naturally arises. The good idea of having independent data monitoring committees of the early 1990s is appearing to go on steroids and resulting confusion for clinicians and their patients is inevitable.

8.9.5 Mergers and Licensing

During the course of a clinical trial, the sponsor could merge or be acquired by another company or the experimental drug could be licensed to another company. This change in ownership of the product might result in immediate personnel changes in the sponsor and there may be a period where it is not clear who is in charge at the sponsor or what the plans are for the continuation of the DMC. The new ownership may have different SOPs for a DMC and safety monitoring than the original owner and the new owner may want to choose their own DMC. In these cases, it is the responsibility of the original DMC to see that the trial is not orphaned. The DMC must make sure that independent stewardship of the trial continues. The DMC Chair will have the responsibility of finding out who is now in charge and what the plans are for safety monitoring. Unfortunately if the new owner says that the original DMC will not be needed and does not disclose its current plans for safety monitoring, there is not much that the DMC can do to correct this matter. A more typical situation is that there is a new sponsor but the original sponsor must continue the safety monitoring until the trial is completed. This orderly transfer makes a lot of sense and is in the best interest of both companies and the patients. The DMC may find that sponsor staff are less interested in the trial now than they were before the change in ownership but the DMC Chair must not allow this change in attitude to affect DMC attitude or commitment.

8.9.6 Journal Policies Regarding Independent Reviews

Recently, *JAMA* published a policy on publication of results of industry-sponsored clinical trials (Fontanarosa, Flanagin, and DeAngelis 2005). The new policy included the inclusion of an independent DMC to oversee the trial. This may have come as no surprise. However, the policy statement also included a requirement that an academic-based biostatistician receives the data from the trial, verifies the appropriateness of the design and analysis plan, and makes an independent analysis of results. There was no mention of what would happen if the sponsor and independent biostatistician results did not agree. This is a very controversial policy and it may never be implemented at least in this form. If there is an independent biostatistical review, DMCs can expect comments on the following types of safety analyses: multiplicity, unplanned analyses, informative censoring and competing risks, assay sensitivity (power), and so on. All of these issues that were covered in Chapters 5 or 6 would not necessarily all wind up in a publication. If comments like these are generated, DMC members will have to meet with sponsor representatives to decide how to proceed.

8.9.7 Fraud Detection

The advent of centralized statistical monitoring as described above is expected to bring data of higher quality to DMCs and provide members with metrics to work with sponsors to focus on clinical sites that need improvement. However, in the process of investigating data inconsistency, it is inevitable that evidence of fraud will be detected. George and Buyse (2015) have written a definitive paper on fraud in clinical trials and George (2016) has provided a scholarly history on research misconduct. He references a meta-analysis by Fanelli (2009) which surveys the literature for data on scholars' awareness of data fabrication, falsification, and other questionable research practice which places the overall percent of studies with misconduct at the astonishing level of 14%. This level is expected to increase due to the considerable pressures to enroll patients on clinical trials and the number of first-time investigators participating in clinical trials in countries that had not been previously involved in industry clinical trials.

Herson (2016) has developed procedures for what sponsors can do to salvage a clinical trial once fraud is detected. Foremost among the procedures is the Fraud Recovery Plan (FRP). This is a plan that would be written before the start of a clinical trial and be administered to both the sponsor and the DMC. The paper provides suggestions of what the FRP might specify in the face of falsification of eligibility criteria, underreporting of adverse events, creation of fictional patients, fabrication of patient diaries, and so on. An important decision would be to just drop the fraudulent data or all the data from the "guilty" site. He addresses the possibility of using imputation methods to replace the fabricated data. Fraud in primary endpoints as well as fraud in important covariates is explored as well as the effect of fraud on randomization, planned interim analysis, and estimation of effect size. Much of the trial can be salvaged if an FRP is put in place before the trial begins. The DMC would approve the FRP prior to the start of the trial and administer the FRP, when necessary, working with both sponsor, regulators, and other entities who may investigate the matter.

8.9.8 Compensation of DMC Members

The question of whether a DMC can be truly independent when the members are recruited and compensated by sponsors has lingered for some time. It may be time to at least experiment with regulators taking over the responsibility of creating DMCs for a particular trial and for compensating them. Clearly FDA recruits and compensates advisory committee members and the NIH recruits and compensates their advisory committees and study sections. The cost of this program could be funded by PDUFA (Prescription Drug User Fee Act) fees. It would attract DMC experts who are willing to work for the modest compensation of government service and to be responsible to the FDA rather than those who prefer to negotiate a fee with the sponsor and who want to identify with a prestigious Big Pharma or exiting Infant Pharma. Most important, this arrangement would keep the regulators in the loop with the sponsor during a clinical trial and it would be possible for the DMC to discuss issues with regulators and advisory committee members on an unmasked basis.

Of course, there would be problems with such an arrangement but an experiment where FDA would randomize drugs of a certain type such as breast cancer, cardiovascular disease, to be developed under the traditional DMC–sponsor organization or the FDA compensation scheme would be helpful. After the trials are completed FDA would compare the results and assess the feasibility of implementing regulator compensation perhaps, initially, only for certain drug classes.

8.10 Resignation from a DMC

It is always hoped that a DMC member will not have to resign during the lifetime of the clinical trial. However, there are, first, some obvious reasons for a member having to resign. These would involve conflicts of interest that have arisen from changes that have taken place since the trial began. Examples would be becoming an investigator in a trial for a competing product, becoming an employee of another pharmaceutical firm, becoming more involved with the sponsor as a consultant, and so on. There are personal reasons such as health and increased workload at one's own institution that would also lead to resignation.

DMC members may have serious disagreements with other DMC members or sponsors that cannot be resolved. These disagreements may be over the nature of data analysis, safety concerns, or ethical issues. There may also be personality conflicts between DMC members or with sponsor representatives. Whatever the reason, the DMC members must be sure that they have heard the problem of the DMC member's concern and done everything to resolve the problem.

The next step after the resignation would be for the DMC to work with the sponsor to see that a qualified replacement is found and, if possible, the resigning member continues to serve until the replacement is in place.

The DMC Charter will typically list criteria for which the sponsor can terminate a DMC member. If this should happen, the procedures of the preceding paragraph would apply.

It should be kept in mind that when a DMC member resigns or is terminated for some type of disagreement, the morale of the other DMC members is likely to be affected and it may take some time to overcome that. The personality and the abilities of the replacement member will be very important in bringing about the recovery needed.

Table 8.3 presents a list of useful items for the Data Review Plan. Table 8.4 displays a list of potential DMC responsibilities arising in this chapter.

TABLE 8.3

Useful Items for the Data Review Plan

1. Details of the DMC role in safety assessment in adaptive designs and other novel designs all of which are efficacy oriented.
2. Will PRO-CTCAE be used?
3. Companion diagnostics—sensitivity, specificity, and predictive accuracy if known at the beginning of trial. If not known what are the targets?
4. Plan for preservation of masking if surrogate endpoint has an unmasking potential.
5. Relationship between Data Monitoring Committee, Steering Committee and Safety Assessment Committee, and the decision-making hierarchy.
6. Details of the Fraud Recovery Plan.

Note: A complete list of useful items for the DRP will be found in Appendix Table A.2.

TABLE 8.4

Potential DMC Responsibilities Arising in This Chapter

Make sure the ability of the DMC to report safety concerns is built into adaptive designs and other novel designs.

Approve any change in effect size of interest taking the current safety profile into account.

In basket trials make sure the DMC has the needed tumor-specific expertise.

Under centralized statistical monitoring keep track of data quality metrics by site and advise the sponsor on needed improvement.

In a SMART/DTS trial make sure that there is adequate safety information for the decision branches of interest.

Make sure that PRO-CTCAE severity data are taken seriously.

For pragmatic trials make sure all members understand that they are working on a pragmatic rather than an efficacy trial.

In biosimilar trials make sure that safety differences are discussed and investigated.

In the event of merger or licensing make sure that patient safety is protected by independent review in the transition plan to the new sponsor.

For companion diagnostics, review the sensitivity, specificity, and predictive accuracy of the diagnostic and make sure that these metrics conform to scientific and industry standards.

Administer the Fraud Recovery Plan when fraud is detected.

For training purposes, if a DMC member resigns for a noncontroversial reason, suggest replacing this person with someone who has not previously served on a DMC.

Note: A complete list of DMC responsibilities will be found in Appendix Table A.3.

Complete lists of DRP items and DMC responsibilities will be found in Appendix Tables A.2 and A.3, respectively.

8.11 In Conclusion

We have now gone through a book devoted to the state of the art and best practices in safety monitoring through DMCs in pharmaceutical industry clinical trials. This chapter has brought to our attention that the art and science of safety monitoring is constantly in flux partly because of changes in technology and partly because of the maturing of the DMC process. Drugs that fail for safety reasons will go back to the planning stages for some rethinking—perhaps a slightly altered molecule or the same molecule in a different formulation, dose, schedule, different patient types, different indications, and so on. For those products that are approved, the safety monitoring process is not over.

There have been many new guidance documents issued in the past 2 years, all shaping the clinical trial and drug approval process. This book has described their effect on DMC operations as much as can be discerned at this time. In the United States, the *21st Century Cures Act* is making its way through Congress. This act directs the FDA to do whatever it takes to speed up the drug approval process and to implement Bayesian statistical methods wherever possible. If this bill becomes a law, there will be many interpretations but it is likely to have even further effects on DMCs. Like Yogi Berra once said "the future is not what it used to be."

As we said in Chapter 1, we really start to learn about the safety process and the risk versus benefit trade-offs of a new drug in the postapproval era. Here, community physicians will voluntarily submit adverse event reports to regulatory agencies and, eventually, thought leaders will be able to write and speak about risk versus benefit. However, the history of any new drug begins with the safety profile determined from clinical trials and the DMC plays a vital role in this process.

DMCounselor

Q8.1 I am a biostatistical member of a DMC for a renal cell carcinoma trial. At the first meeting of our DMC, I had raised questions about an obviously erroneous early termination rule in the protocol and asked that it be revised to a conventional Lan–DeMets stopping rule. There was agreement to make the change. The second meeting was held in Barcelona. It was only necessary for me to spend two nights at the high-end hotel that the sponsor had chosen for this meeting. I wanted to spend a week in Barcelona and asked the sponsor to send me a round trip tickets with departure and return on two consecutive Saturdays but only two nights at the meeting hotel. The sponsor made a reservation for me to stay seven nights at this hotel at their expense and I told them I only wanted to stay two nights at the conference hotel at their expense. I would stay at another hotel at my expense for the remaining 5 days. The change was made. At the meeting, I found that the protocol change, to correct the statistical error in interim analysis, that I had requested had not been made and, when I complained, the sponsor staff said they had no recollection of my request but they saw nothing wrong with the protocol. I continued to complain about the protocol but raised other questions about the safety analysis. Finally, the senior member of the sponsor team asked the group "don't you think we should invite our biostatistician member to the international renal cell carcinoma conference in Tokyo in October? We need another biostatistician there. Of course our company will pay all expenses." My fellow DMC members, all physicians who would be attending this conference on their own funds, surprisingly agreed. I did not respond to this offer. My fellow DMC members showed no interest in the protocol change I proposed even after I explained its statistical errors. After the meeting, I wrote a letter indicating that if the protocol change was not made in 30 days, I would have to resign from this DMC. They made no reply and I sent a letter of resignation. A response from the sponsor accepted my resignation and indicated that I had a different idea of DMC responsibilities than they had. At an ASCO conference some years later, the results of this trial were reported and, sure enough, a physician from the audience questioned the interim stopping rule and other shady aspects of the analysis. Have you ever heard of such a situation?

A No, you have had some novel experiences. I wonder what idea the sponsor had for the DMC responsibilities. The charter should have spelled this out. As you probably know, pharmaceutical companies have made headlines for offering trips to exotic places to practicing physicians as part of their marketing also claiming that the trip is to seek their valuable advice. This sponsor had not addressed your concerns on the protocol and your resignation was appropriate given the shady nature of this sponsor and lack of support from your fellow DMC members. It would have been a big mistake for you to continue to serve, forget about the protocol, and accept the trip to Tokyo. There are some situations that can be fixed. This is not one of them.

Q8.2 I represent the sponsor of a clinical trial in obstetrics medicine. Some of our DMC members are spending a lot of time reading the tables we provide for their periodic meetings, having a lot of ad hoc phone conferences, and are now requiring further tables. This is increasing the cost of DMC operations beyond our budget and we do not see any significant safety issues on this trial. Are we hostage to this DMC because we cannot be trusted to review safety data ourselves?

A No, you are not hostage to the DMC. If the DMC is asking for more work, the Chair should be able to justify this request without unmasking. You have a right to refuse the request or negotiate the request to a reasonable level. This does not take care of the problem of DMC members doing the routine review of tables but taking more hours than you had in your budget. One way to handle this problem would be to pay the DMC members a fixed quarterly fee regardless of the number of meetings and the volume of the work done. Remind the DMC members that they are providing a service for drug development in their specialization. DMC service is not meant to be a lucrative consulting contract. However, if there is concern that circumstances are demanding more work than the quarterly fee will justify then a discussion between sponsor and DMC Chair is appropriate with the latter having to justify these costs. After this conference, the quarterly fee can be increased. This scheme can also be implemented by paying a fixed fee for each face-to-face meeting and teleconference regardless of the amount of preparation necessary.

Q8.3 I am a physician member of a DMC for a clinical trial for an experimental treatment for treatment-resistant tuberculosis. Our DMC just concluded a successful placebo-controlled phase II trial. FDA has granted accelerated approval for the United States but the sponsor is required to run a phase IV commitment controlled trial. The DMC and sponsor are in agreement that such a trial will not get the needed enrollment in the United States because patients there now have access to the newly approved drug through practitioners. The sponsor wants to do the trial in a third-world country where they have no intention of marketing the product if approved. I feel this is immoral. Should I resign?

A There appears to be reason for you to resign on moral grounds but will that change the problem? It just removes you from participating. You and your fellow DMC members might get the sponsor to agree to market the drug in the third-world country or do an active control trial where every patient will get a drug with some potential to help. The problem the sponsor is facing is inherent in the accelerated approval program. Your DMC could encourage the sponsor to talk to FDA about this problem. There may be another way of meeting the phase IV commitment. The sponsor should definitely use your argument about the moral implications of doing a controlled trial of any kind in the third world when the sponsor has a recently approved drug for a serious disease. The sponsor's argument might also be aided by telling FDA that the DMC cannot morally work on such a trial.

Q8.4 I am Chair of a DMC working on an oncology trial for an Infant Pharma company. The DAC responsibilities are being handled by a CRO under contract with the sponsor. The DAC has now stopped work on this project because they are in a dispute regarding overdue payments from the sponsor. The DMC members are frustrated in being in the middle of this dispute and because of the uncertainty over when our next DMC meeting can be held. One member has suggested that we all resign under the justification that "sponsor and DAC deserve one another." Should we do this? What options do we have?

A The first thing to consider when situations like this arise is that the DMC exists to protect patient safety. The DMC should not resign unless suitable arrangements are made for the continuing safety surveillance. Money problems occur often with Infant Pharma but these sponsors know that they must work out their financial and contractor problems as soon as they can because the clinical trials are an important asset. The DAC is under contract with the sponsor but their contract is not like one for cleaning carpets or delivering bottled water. They too have a responsibility for patient safety and they should carefully consider the implications of a work stoppage. Keep your DMC together. This too shall pass.

Q8.5 I am Chair of a DMC working on a lung cancer protocol. In the open session of every meeting, the sponsor gives a long discourse on the uncertainty of whether or not FDA will approve the companion diagnostic they are using on the trial. We already have enrolled 100 patients. The sponsor cannot use a different diagnostic because they do not have a business relationship with another diagnostic company and the other diagnostic company has an exclusive relationship with a sponsor of a competing drug currently in development. During our last closed session, one of our members searched the Internet for the companion diagnostics company and read that the two diagnostic companies are in a patent dispute. Do we, as a DMC, have any responsibility in all of this?

A This whole world of precision medicine and companion diagnostics is causing oncologists to be physicians, biologists, and intellectual property lawyers. The sponsor is doing a good job of including the DMC in their interactions with FDA. The DMC should sympathize with the sponsor on these issues but the DMC responsibility is not to advocate for a companion diagnostic but to review the safety data on the trial and the enrollment levels. Listen patiently to these reports but don't feel that you have a direct role.

Q8.6 I am the biostatistical member of a pragmatic clinical trial for exotic infection experienced by cancer patients. It is a randomized trial with an active control. The trial is being conducted by community physicians with a loose protocol regarding changing dose and schedule. Our Chair is an infectious disease expert and the other physician is an oncologist. The Chair has been taking a lot of time in open session to tell the sponsor that there is a need for a protocol change because the physicians are making irrational decisions and this will mask the efficacy of the drug. I have tried to explain to him that this is a pragmatic trial and how this product works in the community is exactly what we are researching. The oncologist has little to say. How should I handle this?

A Nobody said implementing pragmatic trials with sponsors used to the more traditional trials was going to be easy. You have explained the point correctly. The sponsor should have made a better orientation to your committee explaining the difference between a pragmatic trial and a traditional trial. Of course, even if they had, old habits die hard. I would think that sponsors need to look to community physicians as DMC members for this type of trial. For this trial just hang in there. Perhaps, you and the sponsor can engage the Chair by asking him/her to write guidelines of the use of the product by community physicians after the trial is completed or ask if he/she would like to speak to physician associations in some key cities.

Q8.7 I am the biostatistician member of a DMC working on a prostate cancer protocol. The sponsor added PRO-CTCAE questions for two

AESIs. The two physician members, both oncologists, are saying that the sponsor should ignore the patient AE grading because they have worked on PRO-CTCAE protocols before and the patients tend to guess what treatment they are on and imagine AEs and severity on that basis rather than real experience. I don't know what to make of this. I have not read about this issue in the literature.

A   Well, oncologists have been guessing treatments and reporting AEs accordingly ever since there were double-masked trials in oncology. Why shouldn't patients have a chance? I see no reason for your physician members to be dismissive of the PRO-CTCAE responses. We are in the early days of using this type of data and, for that reason, I don't understand how the physicians can claim so much experience. I think this is just a case of the doctors feeling that defining and grading adverse events is a physician responsibility and only they can do this with the precision required. They should understand that the PRO-CTCAE responses are not replacing the investigator grading. Both will be used and, perhaps, the regulators will take into account that there is not a lot of experience with the patient-reported severity in their safety review. I am sure they will not ignore the data.

Glossary

(Terms are defined within the context of this book rather than more generally.)

active control: The control treatment is an approved drug rather than a placebo (Chapter 6).

adaptive design: A clinical trial design where the trial becomes redesigned due to data collected during the trial, such as changing sample size, dropping a dose group (Chapter 8).

add-on design: A clinical trial design that compares Treatment A with Treatments A + B where A is an approved drug and B is the experimental drug (Chapter 6).

ad hoc consultant: A person appointed to assist a DMC on specific matters involving expertise not present on the DMC such as an allergist being consulted on hypersensitivity on an ophthalmology trial (Chapter 2).

ad hoc meeting: A DMC meeting that had not been previously scheduled but called to discuss a specific recently occurring safety issue (Chapter 3).

adherers: Those patients enrolled in a trial who are complying with the protocol (Chapter 5).

adverse event (AE): An *adverse event* is any unfavorable and unintended sign (e.g., including an abnormal laboratory finding), symptom, or disease temporally associated with the use of a drug, whether or not considered related to the drug. The term *treatment emergent* is often added as a modifier in order to remove manifestations of preexisting conditions from consideration (Chapter 4).

adverse event grade: See **adverse event severity**.

adverse event of special interest (AESI): Adverse event of concern, typically Tier 1 adverse events (Chapter 4).

adverse event severity: A measure of the intensity or extent of the event, sometimes called grade (Chapter 4).

alpha-spending function: In interim analysis the significance levels for hypothesis testing at each planned analysis, for example, O'Brien–Fleming, Lan–DeMets (Chapter 7).

alternative hypothesis: In statistical hypothesis testing the hypothesis that indicates that there is a difference in adverse event incidence between treatment groups (Chapter 5).

APPROVe: Acronym for the Adenomatous Polyp Prevention on Vioxx clinical trial (Chapter 5).

assay sensitivity: A statistical calculation of the magnitude of treatment difference in adverse event incidence that can be detected with the sample sizes in each treatment group (Chapter 5).

attained significance level: See **p-value**.

bad news travels first: A phenomenon in clinical trial communications where data reporting deaths or SAEs arrive at the sponsor before data on routine visits, thus putting these events out of proportion to follow-up time on the trial (Chapter 7).

basket design: In oncology a master protocol design where several drugs are rotated to a genetic mutation regardless of tumor type (Chapter 8).

Bayesian methods: Statistical methods that combine prior information on adverse event incidence with data collected on the clinical trial (Chapter 5).

benefit–risk: See **risk versus benefit**.

bias: An observed treatment difference due to effects other than treatments themselves and/or nonobjective actions in operations or evaluations (Chapter 6).

Big Pharma: A pharmaceutical firm with many products on the market (Chapter 1).

binomial distribution: A statistical distribution used to determine the probability of observing a specified number of adverse events given an assumed adverse event incidence (Chapter 5).

biomarkers: A clinical measurement that is predictive of a future outcome such as a skin rash predicting efficacy in an oncology trial (Chapter 8).

biosimilar designs: A bioequivalence design for follow-on biologics. The biologics analog to generic drugs (Chapter 8).

black box warning: A communication between a regulatory agency and practicing physicians of a very important serious adverse event associated with a drug. The warning is enclosed in a black box on the package insert (Chapter 1).

blinded: Treatment identity is hidden, see also **masked** (Chapter 1).

BRAT—Benefit Risk Action Team: An industry group working on quantification of risk versus benefit (Chapter 7).

case report form (CRF): A form used to collect all of the clinical data during the trial. It should be reviewed by the DMC prior to the outset of the trial (Chapter 4).

category A, B, C: Three types of SUSAR depending on the origin of evidence of causality (Chapter 4).

causal inference: A statistical method that allows conclusions of causation in clinical trials for variables other than treatment group (Chapter 8).

censored observation: In time-to-event analysis the time contribution for a patient who did not experience an adverse event (Chapter 5).

chi square test: A statistical method for assessing the difference in adverse event incidence between treatment groups (Chapter 5).

clinical research associate (CRA): A member of the safety monitoring team who provides site monitoring services (Chapter 1).

companion diagnostic: See *in vitro* **companion diagnostic device**.

CHW method: A method of sample size reestimation (Chapter 8).

Clopper–Pearson confidence interval: See **exact binomial confidence interval**.

closed session: The phase of a DMC meeting where the DMC members and the DAC statistician meet (Chapter 3).

competing risks: A statistical artifact that occurs when the occurrence of one event causes a reduced likelihood of another event. In the context of safety analysis, a treatment group where patients experience early deaths may have less cardiovascular toxicity than a treatment group where patients don't die early but this might just be due to the fact that patients who die early are not treated long enough to develop cardiovascular adverse events (Chapter 6).

conditional power: Given the data at hand at an interim point in a clinical trial the probability of detecting a treatment difference in adverse event incidence at the end of the trial under the assumption of the trajectory of future data (Chapter 7).

confidence interval: A statistical method for estimating a plausible range for adverse event incidence (Chapter 5).

confirmatory trial: Typically, a phase III clinical trial. It is the trial(s) on which regulatory approval will be based. Also called a pivotal trial. Most DMCs are working on confirmatory trials (Chapter 1).

conflict of interest: A situation where a DMC member might not be considered sufficiently independent such as if he/she owns stock in the sponsor or a company offering a competing product. This possibility must be reviewed before a member may be appointed to a DMC (Chapter 2).

contract research organization (CRO): An organization under contract with the sponsor to take over tasks often performed by the sponsor such as site monitoring, report writing, and biostatistics (Chapter 2).

CIOMS form: A form developed by the Council for International Organizations of Medical Sciences that is used for narrative reports of adverse events. It ensures that the history, concomitant medications, preexisting conditions, comorbidity, and so on, are all reported. Copies of CIOMS forms, or a sponsor's own version, are distributed to DMC members for all SAEs (Chapter 4).

covariate: A variable that might affect AE incidence such as treatment or geographic region (Chapter 5).

CTCAE (Common Terminology Criteria for Adverse Events): A classification system like MedDRA developed by the U.S. National Cancer Institute for classifying adverse events in oncology trials sponsored by NCI. Oncology investigators must be trained to use MedDRA in pharmaceutical industry-sponsored trials (Chapter 4).

data analysis center (DAC): The organization with the responsibility for preparing tables, listings, graphs, analyses, and so on, for the DMC.

The DAC will be unmasked so it would have to be a separate independent unit if within the sponsor. The DAC is often found at a contract research organization working under contract with the sponsor. The DAC contributes an independent statistician as a nonvoting member of the DMC (Chapter 2).

data monitoring committee (DMC): A committee created by a sponsor to provide independent review of accumulating safety and efficacy data. This committee is responsible for the stewardship of the trial which translates to protecting trial integrity and patient safety (Chapter 1).

data review meeting: A regular occurring DMC meeting where the DMC will review accumulated safety data (Chapter 3).

data review plan (DRP): The detailed plan for the DMC's data review—tables, listings, graphs, statistical methods, interim analyses, and so on (Chapters 2 through 8).

"Dear Investigator" letter: A letter written by a sponsor to investigators alerting them to unexpected adverse events observed on the trial or asking them to change operations for supportive care, infection control, and so on (Chapter 7).

decision matrix: A table created by a DMC in closed session prior to unmasking indicating the course of action to be followed for various potential distributions of adverse events between treatment groups (Chapter 7).

deductive inference: In medicine, given the disease what symptoms can we expect (Chapter 5).

DMC Charter: A document approved by the sponsor and DMC at the outset of a clinical trial that indicates the scope and rules and regulations of DMC operations (Chapter 2).

double false discovery rate (DFDR): A method of controlling for multiplicity by applying the false discovery rate (FDR) twice (Chapter 5).

drift: At interim analysis, an assumption of the future trajectory of efficacy data (Chapter 7).

drug label: See **package insert**.

effect size: A measure of the difference in an efficacy parameter between experimental and control treatment (Chapter 8).

Elements to Assure Safe Use (ETASU): A specific program within an REMS, risk evaluation, and mitigation strategy (Chapter 3).

endpoint adjudication committee: A masked committee that decides whether or not a patient achieved an efficacy endpoint (Chapter 2).

ethics committee: See **institutional review board**.

evidence: Information gained from a clinical trial on adverse event incidence (Chapter 5).

exact binomial confidence interval: A confidence interval computed on the basis of the binomial distribution rather than the normal distribution (Chapter 5).

executive session: If needed, the phase of a closed session where the DMC members meet without the presence of the DAC statistician (Chapter 3).

expedited SAE: An SAE that is unexpected, regulatory agencies require prompt reporting of this class of SAEs, and they should simultaneously be reported to the DMC (Chapter 4).

exploratory trials: Typically phase I and II clinical trials (Chapter 1).

false discovery rate (FDR): A statistical method for controlling multiplicity by considering the proportion of all hypotheses declared statistically significant where in fact no treatment effect existed (Chapter 5).

false negative: In statistical hypothesis testing concluding that a treatment difference does not exist when, in fact, a difference exists (Chapter 5).

false positive: In statistical hypothesis testing, concluding a treatment difference when, in fact, the difference does not exist (Chapter 5).

familywise error rate (FWER): See **Type I error**.

Final Rule: A 2012 FDA guidance on expedited safety reporting (Chapter 4).

Firewall: An internal sponsor process by which staff members working on the clinical trial remain masked (Chapter 2).

firewall committee: See **pharmacovigilence committee**.

Fisher's exact test: A statistical method similar to a chi square test but using a discrete probability distribution instead of the normal distribution to determine the p-value (Chapter 5).

fraud recovery plan (FRP): A plan made before the start of a trial that indicates what steps will be taken to salvage the trial should evidence of data fraud be found (Chapter 8).

frequentist methods: Traditional statistical methods based on repeated sampling (Chapter 5).

futility analysis: A planned interim analysis of efficacy to assess, under various assumptions of future drift, the probability that the null hypothesis will be rejected at the end of the trial (Chapter 7).

futility analysis, binding: If an interim analysis concludes futility the trial must terminate (Chapter 7).

futility analysis, nonbinding: If an interim analysis concludes futility the trial is not required to terminate (Chapter 7).

grade: See **adverse event severity**.

granularity: A phenomenon that arises in adverse event classification indicating the extent of specificity in preferred terms (Chapter 6).

group sequential designs: A planned interim analysis with at least one hypothesis test for efficacy before the end of the trial (Chapter 7).

Haybittle Peto: An ad hoc alpha-spending function (Chapter 7).

hazard ratio: In time-to-event analysis the ratio of risk of adverse event per unit time in the experimental group to the control group (Chapter 5).

Hollywood model: A management science term for a team brought together for a single purpose never to come together again in the same form. DMC is an example of the Hollywood model (Chapter 2).

incidence, percent: Proportional incidence × 100% (Chapter 5).

incidence, proportional: The ratio of the number of patients experiencing an adverse event to the total number of patients randomized to that treatment group (Chapter 5).

incomplete observation: See **censored observation**.

Indemnification: A provision in a DMC member's contract whereby the sponsor pledges to hold DMC members against liability issues that may arise in the trial that are not their fault (Chapter 2).

inductive incidence: In medicine, given the symptoms what disease can we expect? (Chapter 5).

independent statistician: A statistician employed by the DAC who will serve as a nonvoting member of the DMC and unmask the DMC members if requested (Chapter 2).

Infant Pharma: A pharmaceutical firm with no revenues from product sales and no products on the market (Chapter 1).

information time: The proportion of patients who have completed a trial, for time-to-event endpoints the proportion of patients who have had an event, and the denominator being the total number of events not the total number of patients (Chapter 7).

informed consent: A document prepared by the institution performing a clinical trial in which it informs potential patient volunteers, among other things, of possible adverse events they might experience in the trial (Chapter 3).

institutional review board (IRB): In the United States a committee that exists at every institution performing research on human subjects. The committee reviews all aspects of the research in order to protect the safety of human subjects. Similar committees in other countries are called ethics committees (Chapter 2).

integrated summary of safety (ISS): A section of a new drug application that summarizes safety data for the experimental treatment over all human trials. It should be established at the DMC orientation meeting if the DMC will be expected to review the ISS prior to submission to the regulatory agency (Chapter 3).

internal safety review committee (ISRC): A group of sponsor employees not working on the clinical trial of interest performing a function in parallel with a DMC (Chapter 8).

International Conference on Harmonisation (ICH): A joint effort between the United States, Europe, and Japan to create international agreement on regulations for the approval of new drugs (Chapter 1).

investigator brochure: A document prepared by the sponsor before the trial begins that summarizes all known information about the experimental drug used in the trial. It should be reviewed by the DMC at the outset of a trial (Chapter 3).

investigator-sponsored trial: An experimental clinical trial where the investigator takes on all responsibilities for reporting progress and adverse events to a regulatory agency (Chapter 1).

in vitro **companion diagnostic device:** A diagnostic used to screen patients for a biomarker before entry to a clinical trial (Chapter 8).

Kaplan–Meier graph: A statistical method of graphically depicting the cumulative frequency of adverse events over time (Chapter 5).

lambda (λ): The parameter (mean) of the Poisson distribution (Chapter 5).

Lan–DeMets design: A group sequential design (Chapter 7).

landmark estimate: In time-to-event analysis the estimate of adverse event incidence at a particular point in time such as 12 months after treatment start (Chapter 5).

learning trials: See **exploratory trials**.

likelihood function: An expression giving the degree of belief in various levels of adverse event incidence conditional on the data observed in the trial (Chapter 5).

likelihood graph: A graph showing the relative likelihood for each value of adverse event incidence (Chapter 5).

likelihood methods: Statistical methods based on the data already collected rather than repeated sampling (Chapter 5).

log rank test: A statistical method for determining the p-value for the difference between treatment groups in a time-to-event/Kaplan–Meier analysis (Chapter 5).

logistic regression analysis: A multifactor method to assess the influence of covariate factors on AE incidence and compute adjusted rates (Chapter 5).

masked: Treatment identity is hidden. Synonym for blinded but used here to avoid confusion in ophthalmology clinical trials (Chapter 1).

masked, partially: A policy whereby DMC members know the treatments as A, B, C, and so on, but do not know the identity of the treatment codes (Chapter 5).

MedDRA—medical dictionary for regulatory affairs: A system for coding adverse events that is generally used in pharmaceutical industry clinical trials (Chapter 4).

medical governance committee: See **pharmacovigilence committee**.

meta-analysis: A statistical method for bringing together data from previous clinical trials in an effort to create one combined estimate of effect size or adverse event incidence (Chapter 7).

meta-analysis, APD: Aggregate patient data, see **meta-analysis, retrospective** (Chapter 7).

meta-analysis, fixed effects: The treatment effect being estimated is assumed to be fixed across trials (Chapter 7).

meta-analysis, IPD: Individual patient data, see **meta-analysis, prospective** (Chapter 7).

meta-analysis, prospective: Performed on patient-level data from various trials (Chapter 7).

meta-analysis, random effects: The treatment effect being estimated is assumed to vary randomly across trials (Chapter 7).

meta-analysis, retrospective: Performed on data extracted from the literature (Chapter 7).

Middle Pharma: A pharmaceutical firm with one or two recently approved products on the market (Chapter 1).

monitoring, safety: Continual review of accumulating safety data during a clinical trial (Chapter 1).

monitoring, site: A quality control procedure applied periodically during the trial by sponsor or contract clinical research associates (Chapter 1).

monitoring, centralized risk based: Algorithm methods for assessing data quality as opposed to site monitoring by clinical research associates (Chapter 8).

monitoring, statistical: Making calculations on accumulating efficacy data to justify early termination of a clinical trial (Chapter 1).

multiplicity: The statistical phenomenon where many tests of hypothesis increase the probability of false positive results (Chapter 5).

NNH (number needed to harm): As how many patients would have to be treated with the experimental treatment to observe an additional adverse event compared to control treatment (Chapter 7).

NNH/NNT ratio: A "quick and dirty" estimate of risk–benefit. It is the number of unfavorable events are prevented by the experimental treatment for each AE caused (Chapter 7).

NNT (number needed to treat): The number of patients that would have to be treated with the experimental treatment to prevent an additional unfavorable event (death, disease progression, nonresponse, etc.) compared to control treatment (Chapter 7).

noninferiority trial: A clinical trial that has its objective to show that an experimental treatment is no worse than active control and possibly superior (Chapter 8).

null hypothesis: In statistical hypothesis testing the hypothesis that there is no difference in adverse event incidence between treatment groups (Chapter 5).

O'Brien–Fleming Design: A group sequential design (Chapter 7).

odds ratio: A measure of relative risk of adverse event in experimental treatment group to control group (Chapter 5).

one-sided test: A statistical hypothesis test that considers whether adverse event incidence in the experimental treatment group is statistically significantly greater than in control group (Chapter 5).

open label: Opposite of masked, treatment identity is known (Chapter 1).

open label extension studies: A follow-up program where patients exit a clinical trial but continue on the experimental treatment for an uncontrolled phase in order to gather long-term safety data. Often used in neurology and oncology (Chapter 1).

open session: The first phase of a DMC meeting where the sponsor staff, DAC members, and DMC members meet to discuss trial progress and report on issues of interest to all (Chapter 3).

orientation (organizational) meeting: The first meeting between the DMC, DAC, and the sponsor staff (Chapter 3).

p-value: The probability that a treatment difference could have occurred due to chance if, in fact, there was no population difference in treatments (Chapter 5).

package insert: Sometimes called the drug label, the document prepared by the sponsor that provides all prescribing information to the physician including adverse events. It should be established at the DMC orientation meeting whether or not the DMC will be responsible for reviewing the proposed package insert prior to submission to the regulatory agency (Chapter 3).

pharmacovigilence staff: A group of sponsor employees separated from the clinical trial staff by a "firewall" charged with reviewing adverse events, possibly unmasked, during the trial. They may call matters of concern to the attention of the DMC (Chapter 4).

pharmacovigilence committee: A committee of sponsor staff not involved in the clinical trial to whom the DMC can consult with if they have a serious safety concern. This avoids unmasking the sponsor staff working on the trial. It is sometimes called a firewall committee or medical governance committee (Chapter 3).

phase I trial: Early safety trial, DMCs are not usually involved (Chapter 1).

phase II trial: Safety trial to refine dose and early efficacy trial, DMCs are sometimes involved (Chapter 1).

pivotal trial: The trial(s) on which regulatory approval will be based, also called a confirmatory trial, typically phase III. Most DMCs are working on pivotal trials (Chapter 1).

planned interim analysis: A protocol-directed time when an analysis for early termination for efficacy, futility, or sample size reestimation will occur (Chapter 7).

Poisson distribution: A probability distribution for rare adverse events based on a mean per time unit (Chapter 5).

Poisson rate ratio: The ratio of rate/100 patient years in experimental treatment group to control group (Chapter 5).

posterior distribution: In Bayesian statistical analysis the probability distribution of adverse event incidence that results when the prior distribution is combined with the distribution of data collected in the clinical trial (Chapter 5).

postmarket surveillance: The process of monitoring incidence of adverse events after a drug has been approved, usually performed by forms being submitted to the sponsor by practicing physicians (Chapter 1).

power: In statistical hypothesis testing the probability that the null hypothesis of no treatment difference will be rejected when the treatments, in fact, differ given the sample size in each group (Chapter 5).

pragmatic trial: An effectiveness rather than efficacy trial where patients are randomized to treatments but clinicians are free to apply those treatments and respond to adverse events any way they feel best (Chapter 8).

predictive power: The Bayesian analog to conditional power (Chapter 7).

preferred term (PT): In MedDRA a term within a system order class (SOC) to describe a specific adverse event, for example, within cardiovascular, myocardial infarct (Chapter 4).

PRISMA statement (Preferred Reporting Items for Systematic Reviews and Meta-Analysis): A checklist of items that should be included in a meta-analysis report (Chapter 7).

progression-free survival: In oncology trials a patient is defined as a treatment failure if he/she experiences progression of disease or dies from any cause, whichever occurs first (Chapter 6).

prior distribution: In Bayesian statistical analysis a probability distribution describing prior beliefs in adverse event incidence distribution (Chapter 5).

PRO-CTCAE: In oncology trials an adverse event severity scale based on patient-reported severity rather than investigator-reported severity (Chapter 8).

program safety analysis plan (PSAP): The elements of safety analysis to be used for the sponsor data analysis during and at the end of the trial. The data review plan (DRP) is a similar document for DMC operations (Chapter 3).

proof of concept: A term usually used in patent law. It is used here to describe a preclinical study or an early phase clinical trial (Chapter 1).

publication bias: A phenomenon that occurs when a clinical trial with a positive result is more likely to be published than one with negative results (Chapter 7).

rate/100 patient years: Computed as the number of patients experiencing an adverse event × 100 divided by the total patient years contributed by that treatment group (Chapter 5).

regulator's risk: In efficacy analysis, another term for Type I error (Chapter 5).

relative risk: A comparison of adverse event incidence between treatment groups. Similar to odds ratio (Chapter 5).

reverse Kaplan–Meier: A method of evaluating the efficiency of patient follow-up (Chapter 5).

risk-based monitoring: A data quality procedure that replaces routine site monitoring by clinical research associates (Chapter 4).

risk–benefit: See **risk versus benefit**.

risk evaluation and mitigation strategies (REMS): A plan drafted by the sponsor that provides steps to be taken to minimize the effect of adverse events of concern such as special training for physicians and requiring certain laboratory tests (Chapter 3).

risk versus benefit: Trade-off between safety and efficacy (Chapter 4).

reconsenting: A process whereby, due to the discovery of unexpected adverse events, patients are asked to sign a revised informed consent form (Chapter 7).

run-in screening phase: A prerandomization phase of a clinical trial where prospective patients must qualify for the trial by, for example, recording a sufficient number of seizures or having a diastolic blood pressure within a certain range (Chapter 5).

safety assessment committee: A committee of physicians, biostatisticians, epidemiologists, and so on, formed by a sponsor to investigate emerging safety concerns through literature search, data from other clinical trials, preclinical studies, and so on (Chapter 1).

safety monitoring: See **monitoring, safety.**

safety monitoring plan (SMP): A document prepared by the sponsor at the outset of a clinical trial indicating responsibilities and procedures for the DMC, DAC, sponsor pharmacovigilence staff, investigators, clinical research associates, and so on. It should be reviewed by the DMC at the outset of a trial (Chapter 3).

safety monitoring team: A term used to encompass all persons and organizations involved with the monitoring of safety during a clinical trial. It would include the sponsor clinical research and pharmacovigilence staffs, CRO staff, DMC members, DAC, and so on (Chapter 2).

sample size reestimation: At planned interim analysis, increase the sample size in order to increase power to reject null hypothesis at the end of the trial (Chapter 8).

screen failure rate: The percentage of patients who do not pass the run-in screening phase of a trial (Chapter 5).

screening phase: See **run-in screening phase.**

seamless transition, phase II to phase III: An adaptive design where a phase II trial becomes a phase III trial after certain conditions are satisfied and the phase II data are used as part of the phase III trial (Chapter 8).

serious adverse event (SAE): Any untoward medical occurrence that, at any dose, results in death, is life-threatening, requires inpatient hospitalization or prolongation of existing hospitalization, results in persistent or significant disability/incapacity, or is a congenital anomaly/birth defect. This is both a clinical and regulatory term (Chapter 4).

Severity: See **adverse event severity.**

significance level: A pretrial setting of the p-value that will determine statistical significance, often p-value less than 0.05 (Chapter 5).

site monitoring: See **monitoring, site.**

SMART/DTS trial designs: Sequential multiple assignment randomization trial or dynamic treatment strategy trial where patients are randomized to one of several protocol-directed treatments at each decision point in the trial (Chapter 8).

SPERT: Safety Planning, Evaluation, and Reporting Team, a pharmaceutical industry group that made suggested procedures for safety analysis (Chapter 4).

solicited adverse event collection: Under this method patients respond to a prepared list of adverse events on each clinic visit (Chapter 6).

sponsor: The organization that has the ultimate responsibility for reporting the results to the regulatory authorities. For our purposes it will most often be a pharmaceutical or biotechnology company but it could be a university, government agency, or, in the case of orphan drugs, a patient–parent support group (Chapter 1).

sponsor representative: The employee of the sponsor who will serve as the liaison with the DMC (Chapter 2).

sponsor's risk: In efficacy analysis, another term for Type II error (Chapter 5).

spontaneous adverse event collection: On a clinic visit the clinician asks the patient if they have had any side effects since last visit (Chapter 6).

statistical monitoring: See **monitoring, statistical**.

standard operating procedures (SOPs): Written procedures used by a sponsor covering all clinical operations, this should include procedures for the formation and operation of a DMC (Chapter 2).

standardized MedDRA queries (SMQ): Combinations of MedDRA preferred terms across system organ classes created to reduce granularity (Chapter 4).

statistical analysis plan (SAP): A document prepared before the start of a clinical trial indicating all definitions, assumptions, and methods for the analysis of data at the conclusion of the trial (Chapter 3).

steering committee: A committee that advises the sponsor on overall trial operations (Chapter 2).

Stewardship: The act of providing careful and responsible management of something entrusted in one's care. The term is said here to describe the overall responsibility of a DMC (Chapter 1).

superiority trial: A clinical trial whose objective is to show that the experimental treatment is superior in efficacy to control (Chapter 8).

support limits: The likelihood analog of confidence interval, a range of plausible values of adverse event incidence, or relative risk (Chapter 5).

SUSAR: Serious Unexpected Suspected Adverse Reactions—a sponsor designation of an unexpected severe AE being causally related to the experimental drug. Expedited reporting required (Chapter 4).

system organ class (SOC): MedDRA is a hierarchical adverse event classification system. The SOC is the highest order—gastrointestinal, nervous system, cardiovascular system, and so on (Chapter 4).

test of concept: See **proof of concept**.

theta (θ): The Poisson rate ratio (Chapter 5).

Tier 1 adverse events: A list of AEs for which specific hypotheses and analysis methods are described before the trial begins; adverse events of special interest (Chapter 4).

Tier 2 adverse events: AEs that were not prespecified but have become apparent in safety monitoring in this trial and where there are a sufficient number of events for data analysis (Chapter 4).

Tier 3 adverse events: AEs that were not prespecified but have become apparent in safety monitoring in this trial and where there are a sufficient number of events for data analysis (Chapter 4).

time-to-event analysis: A statistical method that takes into consideration the time to the onset of adverse events. See also **Kaplan–Meier graph** (Chapter 5).

treatment emergent: A modifier for adverse events used to remove manifestations of preexisting conditions from consideration (Chapter 4).

21st Century Cures Act: In the United States a bill making its way through Congress that mandates that FDA supports a more efficient means of drug development (Chapter 8).

two-sided test: A statistical hypothesis test that considers whether adverse event incidence in the experimental treatment group is either statistically significantly greater than control or statistically significantly less than control (Chapter 5).

Type I error: In statistical hypothesis testing the probability that the null hypothesis of no treatment difference is rejected when the null hypothesis is true (Chapter 5).

Type II error—1: Power or the probability that the null hypothesis is not rejected when false (Chapter 5).

umbrella design: In oncology a master protocol design for a single tumor type but several experimental drugs each targeted to patients with a specific biomarker or genetic mutation (Chapter 8).

unmasking, de facto: Persons working on a clinical trial are unmasked to treatment group by observing differences in adverse event frequency, differential visit schedules, or different procedures at visits between treatment groups (Chapter 6).

unmasking, deliberate: A DMC asks the independent statistician to unmask them (Chapter 6).

white space: A term used by adaptive design planners to indicate a period of time when analysis and planning takes place prior to an adaptation of the trial (Chapter 8)

Appendix

TABLE A.1

Incidence of Selected Adverse Events for Approved Drugs in Placebo-Controlled Clinical Trials

Indication	Drug	Class/Type	Selected Adverse Events	Drug Incidence (%) [95% CI]	Placebo Incidence (%) [95% CI]	Odds Ratio [95% CI]
Allergic rhinitis, seasonal	Fexofenadine	Antihistamine	Viral infection	n=679 2.5 [1.5, 4.0]	n=671 1.5 [0.7, 2.7]	1.7 [0.7, 4.2]
			Nausea	1.6 [0.8, 2.9]	1.5 [0.7, 2.7]	1.1 [0.4, 2.9]
			Dysmeno-rrhea	1.5 [0.7, 2.7]	0.3 [0.04, 1.1]	5 [1.1, 47.1]
			Drowsiness	1.5 [0.7, 2.7]	0.3 [0.04, 1.1]	5 [1.1, 47.1]
			Dyspepsia	1.3 [0.6, 2.5]	0.6 [0.2, 2.5]	2.2 [0.6, 10.0]
Arthritis, rheumatoid	Etanercept	TNF receptor blocker	Injection site reaction	n=349 37.0 [31.8, 42.3]	n=152 10.0 [5.6, 15.8]	5.4 [3.0, 10.2]
			Infection	35.0 [30.0, 40.2]	32.0 [24.9, 40.3]	1.1 [0.7, 1.7]
			Headache	17.0 [13.3, 21.3]	13.0 [8.8, 20.1]	1.3 [0.8, 2.5]
			Rhinitis	12.0 [8.8, 15.9]	8.0 [4.1, 13.4]	1.6 [0.8, 3.4]
			Nausea	9.0 [6.1, 12.4]	10.0 [5.6, 15.8]	0.9 [0.5, 1.8]
Cardio-vascular	Ramipril	ACE inhibitor	Hypotension	n=1004 11.0 [9.1, 13.1]	n=982 5.0 [3.7, 6.5]	2.3 [1.7, 3.3]
			Cough	8.0 [6.4, 19.8]	4.0 [2.8, 5.4]	2.1 [1.4, 3.1]
			Dizziness	4.0 [2.9, 5.4]	3.0 [2.0, 4.2]	1.4 [0.8, 2.2]
			Angina pectoris	3.0 [2.0, 4.2]	2.0 [1.2, 3.1]	1.5 [0.8, 2.6]
			Nausea	2.0 [1.2, 3.1]	1.0 [0.5, 1.9]	2.0 [0.9, 4.2]
Cardio-vascular	Metoprolol	Beta-blocker	Hypotension	n=700 27.4 [24.2, 30.9]	n=700 23.2 [20.0, 26.5]	1.3 [1.0, 1.6]
			Heart failure	27.5 [24.2, 30.9]	29.6 [26.2, 33.1]	0.9 [0.7, 1.1]

(Continued)

TABLE A.1 (*Continued*)

Incidence of Selected Adverse Events for Approved Drugs in Placebo-Controlled Clinical Trials

Indication	Drug	Class/Type	Selected Adverse Events	Drug Incidence (%) [95% CI]	Placebo Incidence (%) [95% CI]	Odds Ratio [95% CI]
			Bradycardia	15.9 [13.2, 18.8]	6.7 [5.0, 8.8]	2.6 [1.8, 3.8]
			Heart blockage, 1st degree	5.3 [3.7, 7.2]	1.9 [1.0, 3.2]	2.9 [1.5, 6.1]
			Heart blockage, 2nd or 3rd degree	4.7 [3.3, 6.6]	4.7 [3.3, 6.6]	1.0 [0.6, 1.7]
Depressive disorder, major	Venlafaxine	Anti-depressant	Insomnia	n = 357 17.0 [13.3, 21.4]	n = 285 11.0 [7.5, 15.1]	1.7 [1.0, 2.8]
			Nervousness	10.0 [7.2, 13.7]	5.0 [2.7, 8.1]	2.2 [1.1, 4.4]
			Anorexia	8.0 [5.5, 11.5]	2.0 [0.8, 4.5]	4.1 [1.6, 12.3]
			Weight loss (>5%)	7.0 [4.8, 10.2]	2.0 [0.8, 4.5]	3.5 [1.4, 10.6]
	Paroxetine	Psychotropic	Nausea	n = 421 26.0 [21.8, 30.4]	n = 421 9.0 [6.5, 12.2]	3.5 [2.3, 5.4]
			Somnolence	23.0 [19.1, 27.4]	9.0 [6.5, 12.2]	3.0 [2.0, 4.6]
			Asthenia	15.0 [11.7, 18.7]	6.0 [3.9, 8.6]	2.8 [1.7, 4.7]
			Constipation	14.0 [10.8, 17.7]	9.0 [6.5, 12.2]	1.6 [1.0, 2.6]
			Diarrhea	12.0 [9.2, 15.6]	8.0 [5.7, 11.1]	1.6 [1.0, 2.6]
Diabetes mellitus, type II	Rosiglitazone	Thiazoli-dinedione	Upper respiratory infection	n = 2526 9.9 [8.8, 11.1]	n = 601 8.7 [6.5, 11.2]	1.2 [0.8, 1.6]
			Injury	7.6 [6.6, 8.7]	4.3 [2.8, 6.3]	1.8 [1.2, 2.9]
			Headache	5.9 [5.0, 6.9]	5.0 [3.3, 7.1]	1.2 [0.8, 1.9]
			Back pain	4.0 [3.3, 4.8]	3.8 [2.4, 5.7]	1.0 [0.7, 1.7]
			Hyper-glycemia	3.9 [3.2, 4.8]	5.7 [3.9, 7.8]	0.7 [0.5, 1.0]
Duodenal ulcer, active	Omeprazole	Benzimidazole	Headache	n = 465 6.9 [4.8, 9.6]	n = 64 6.3 [1.7, 15.2]	1.1 [0.4, 4.5]

(Continued)

TABLE A.1 (*Continued*)

Incidence of Selected Adverse Events for Approved Drugs in Placebo-Controlled Clinical Trials

Indication	Drug	Class/Type	Selected Adverse Events	Drug Incidence (%) [95% CI]	Placebo Incidence (%) [95% CI]	Odds Ratio [95% CI]
			Diarrhea	3.0 [1.7, 5.0]	3.1 [0.4, 10.8]	1.0 [0.2, 8.9]
			Abdominal pain	2.4 [1.2, 4.2]	3.1 [0.4, 10.8]	0.8 [0.2, 7.1]
			Nausea	2.2 [1.0, 3.9]	3.1 [0.4, 10.8]	0.7 [0.1, 6.5]
			Upper respiratory infection	1.9 [0.9, 3.6]	1.6 [0.04, 8.4]	1.2 [0.2, 55.4]
Epilepsy	Oxcar-bazepine	Antiepileptic	Vomiting	n = 126 36.0 [27.4, 44.7]	n = 166 5.0 [2.1, 9.3]	11.0 [4.8, 28.0]
			Nausea	29.0 [21.6, 38.1]	10.0 [6.1, 15.9]	3.6 [1.9, 7.3]
			Fatigue	15.0 [9.3, 22.5]	7.0 [3.8, 12.2]	2.3 [1.0, 5.4]
			Abdominal pain	11.0 [6.2, 17.9]	5.0 [2.1, 9.3]	2.5 [0.9, 7.0]
			Diarrhea	7.0 [3.3, 13.1]	6.0 [2.9, 10.8]	1.2 [0.4, 3.4]
Erectile dysfunction	Sildenafil	Sexual dysfunction	Headache	n = 734 16.0 [13.4, 18.8]	n = 725 4.0 [2.7, 5.7]	4.6 [3.0, 7.2]
			Flushing	10.0 [7.8, 12.3]	1.0 [0.4, 2.0]	11.3 [5.2, 29.3]
			Dyspepsia	7.0 [5.2, 9.0]	2.0 [1.2, 3.4]	3.5 [1.9, 6.8]
			Nasal congestion	4.0 [2.7, 5.6]	2.0 [1.2, 3.4]	1.9 [1.0, 3.9]
			Urinary tract infection	3.0 [1.9, 4.5]	2.0 [1.2, 3.4]	1.5 [0.7, 3.1]
Fibro-myalgia	Pregabalin	Neuro-transmitter	Dizziness	n = 600 45.0 [41.0, 49.1]	n = 505 9.0 [6.6, 11.7]	8.3 [5.9, 12.1]
			Somnolence	22.0 [18.8, 25.5]	4.0 [2.4, 6.1]	6.8 [4.2, 11.8]
			Weight increase	14.0 [11.3, 17.0]	2.0 [1.6, 3.6]	8.1 [4.1, 17.6]
			Vision, blurred	12.0 [9.5, 14.9]	1.0 [0.3, 23.0]	13.6 [5.5, 43.6]
			Edema, peripheral	9.0 [6.8, 11.6]	2.0 [1.0, 3.6]	4.9 [2.4, 10.9]

(Continued)

TABLE A.1 (*Continued*)

Incidence of Selected Adverse Events for Approved Drugs in Placebo-Controlled Clinical Trials

Indication	Drug	Class/Type	Selected Adverse Events	Drug Incidence (%) [95% CI]	Placebo Incidence (%) [95% CI]	Odds Ratio [95% CI]
Hypercho-lestero-lemia	Atorvastatin	Lipid lowering	Dry mouth	9.0 [6.8, 11.6]	2.0 [1.0, 3.6]	4.9 [2.4, 10.9]
			Infection	n=863 10.3 [8.4, 12.5]	n=270 10.0 [6.7, 14.2]	1.0 [0.6, 1.7]
			Headache	5.4 [4.0, 7.2]	7.0 [4.3, 10.8]	0.8 [0.4, 1.4]
			Rash	3.9 [2.7, 5.5]	0.7 [0.1, 2.7]	5.5 [1.4, 47.5]
			Abdominal pain	2.8 [1.8, 4.1]	0.7 [0.1, 2.7]	3.8 [0.9, 33.7]
			Back pain	2.8 [1.8, 4.1]	3.0 [1.3, 5.8]	0.9 [0.4, 2.4]
Osteo-porosis	Risedronate	Bisphos-phonate	Arthralgia	n=1914 21.1 [19.3, 23.0]	n=1916 23.7 [21.8, 25.7]	0.9 [0.7, 1.0]
			Abdominal pain	11.6 [10.2, 13.1]	9.4 [8.1, 10.8]	1.3 [1.0, 1.6]
			Urinary tract infection	10.9 [9.5, 12.4]	9.7 [8.4, 11.1]	1.1 [0.9, 1.4]
			Hyper-tension	10.0 [8.7, 11.4]	9.0 [7.7, 10.4]	1.1 [0.9, 1.4]
			Joint disorder	6.8 [5.7, 8.0]	5.4 [4.4, 6.5]	1.3 [1.0, 1.7]
	Teriparatide	Recombinant human parathyroid hormone	Arthralgia	n=691 10.1 [8.0, 12.6]	n=691 8.4 [6.4, 10.7]	1.2 [0.8, 1.8]
			Rhinitis	9.6 [7.5, 12.0]	8.8 [6.8, 11.2]	1.1 [0.7, 1.6]
			Nausea	8.5 [6.4, 10.7]	6.7 [4.9, 8.8]	1.3 [0.8, 2.0]
			Dizziness	8.0 [6.1, 10.2]	5 [3.8, 7.3]	1.5 [1.0, 2.4]
			Hyper-tension	7.1 [5.3, 10.3]	6.8 [5.0, 8.9]	1.0 [0.7, 1.6]
Platelet reduction	Clopidogrel	Adenosine inhibitor	Headache	n=9599 7.6 [7.1, 8.1]	n=9586[a] 7.2 [6.9, 7.7]	1.1 [1.0, 1.2]
			Arthralgia	6.3 [5.8, 6.8]	6.2 [5.7, 6.7]	1.0 [0.9, 1.1]
			Diarrhea	4.5 [4.1, 4.9]	3.4 [3.0, 3.8]	1.3 [1.2, 1.6]

(*Continued*)

TABLE A.1 (*Continued*)

Incidence of Selected Adverse Events for Approved Drugs in Placebo-Controlled Clinical Trials

Indication	Drug	Class/Type	Selected Adverse Events	Drug Incidence (%) [95% CI]	Placebo Incidence (%) [95% CI]	Odds Ratio [95% CI]
			Hyper-tension	4.3 [3.9, 4.7]	5.1 [4.7, 5.6]	0.8 [0.7, 1.0]
			Nausea	3.4 [3.0, 3.8]	3.8 [3.4, 4.2]	0.9 [0.8, 1.0]
Renal failure, chronic	Epoetin	Glycoprotein	Hyper-tension	n = 200 24.0 [18.3, 30.5]	n = 135 19.0 [13.0, 26.9]	1.3 [0.8, 2.4]
			Headache	16.0 [11.2, 21.8]	12.0 [6.9, 18.5]	1.4 [0.7, 2.9]
			Arthralgia	11.0 [7.0, 16.2]	6.0 [2.6, 11.3]	2.0 [0.8, 5.3]
			Nausea	11.0 [7.0, 16.2]	9.0 [4.7, 15.0]	1.3 [0.6, 2.9]
			Edema	9.0 [5.4, 13.9]	10.0 [5.8, 16.8]	0.9 [0.4, 1.9]
Sleep disorder	Eszopiclone	Nonbenzodia-zepine hypnotic agent	Unpleasant taste	n = 105 34.0 [25.3, 44.2]	n = 99 3.0 [0.6, 8.6]	16.7 [4.9, 87.1]
			Headache	17.0 [10.5, 25.7]	13.0 [7.2, 21.4]	1.4 [0.6, 3.2]
			Respiratory infection	10.0 [5.3, 18.0]	3.0 [0.6, 8.6]	3.7 [0.9, 21.4]
			Somnolence	8.0 [3.3, 14.5]	3.0 [0.6, 8.6]	2.6 [0.6, 15.8]
			Dizziness	7.0 [2.7, 13.3]	4.0 [1.1, 10.0]	1.7 [0.4, 8.1]

Source (raw data):   U.S. Food and Drug Administration. 2008c. https://www.accessdata.fda.gov/scripts/cder/drugsatfda/

Note: This material is presented to illustrate material in the text. It is not a substitute for official, professional, and consumer information on these drugs.

[a] Control group received aspirin, not placebo.

TABLE A.2

Items for Inclusion in the Data Review Plan (DRP)

Organizational

Details of SAE data flow

Expected patient accrual graph, expected rate of screen failures

Goals for enrollment of minority patients

Method of transmitting data review materials to DMC members

Unmasked sponsor group or individual DMC contacts when safety concern arises

Will site monitoring or centralizes statistical monitoring be used

Estimated time from data cutoff to DMC meeting

Data review meeting frequency

Frequency of face-to-face meetings

Use of telephone/WebEx for meetings

Clinical

Adverse event dictionary—(most likely MedDRA)

If oncology trial what will be the role of CTCAE

Standardized and proprietary MedDRA queries to be used (SMQs)

Severity grading dictionary to be used

Sample AE narrative form (CIOMS or sponsor proprietary)

Tier 1 adverse events—adverse events of special interest

Tier 2, 3 adverse events added as trial progresses

Data flow of AEs requiring expedited reporting—see Table 3.2

Procedure for creating and updating the SUSAR list—Categories A, B, and C

Particular issues in multiregional trials

Statistical

Shell tables, listings, graphs to be provided, updated as trial progresses

Statistical methods for comparing adverse event frequency or laboratory values between treatment groups
  a. Hypothesis testing
  b. Confidence intervals

Criteria for extreme laboratory values to require AE designation

Correction for multiplicity and/or assay sensitivity calculations in making safety comparisons

Extent of use of likelihood and/or Bayesian method

Minimization of Bias and Pitfalls

List which AEs are collected by solicited method. Assume all others are spontaneous reporting

Note competing risk issues, update as observed

Decision Making

Will there be a formal analysis of risk vs. benefit?

(Continued)

TABLE A.2 (*Continued*)

Items for Inclusion in the Data Review Plan (DRP)

Details of the planned interim analysis:
   a. Tables and graphs
   b. Statistical methods and boundaries
   c. Early termination for efficacy
   d. Early termination for futility (binding or nonbinding)
   e. Conditional power analysis
   f. Sample size reestimation

Emerging Issues

Details of the DMC role in safety assessment in adaptive designs and other novel designs all of which are efficacy oriented

Will PRO-CTCAE be used

Companion diagnostics—sensitivity, specificity, and predictive accuracy if known at beginning of trial. If not known what are the targets?

Plan for preservation of masking if surrogate endpoint has an unmasking potential

Relationship between Data Monitoring Committee, Steering Committee, Safety Assessment Committee, and the decision-making hierarchy

Details of the Fraud Recovery Plan

TABLE A.3

Comprehensive List of Potential DMC Responsibilities

Organizational

Comment on and approve charter

Comment on and approve initial Data Review Plan (DRP)

Comment on protocol and investigator brochure

Comment on informed consent form and subsequent changes

Comment on and suggest changes to SAE data flow

Clarify role of DMC in:
   • Design of integrated summary of safety
   • Manuscripts/publications
   • Risk evaluation and mitigation strategies (REMS)
   • Package insert

Make sure the relationship of the DMC, Steering Committee, Internal Safety Review Committee, and Safety Assessment Committee are understood by all

Clinical

DMC members should decide on being partially masked or unmasked

Clarify Tier 1 adverse events or AESIs (adverse events of special interest)

Approve initial SUSAR (Serious Unexpected Suspected Adverse Reactions) list and establish mechanisms for DMC's role in updating

Periodic data review following DRP (Data Review Plan) and amend as needed

Comment on:
   • Adverse events of concern
   • Enrollment issues

(*Continued*)

TABLE A.3 (*Continued*)

Comprehensive List of Potential DMC Responsibilities

- Screen failure rate
- Minority enrollment
- In multiregional trials—list regional issues of concern

Statistical

Approve formats of tables, listings, and graphs, and statistical methods in the DRP, revise as needed

Comment on enrollment progress

Comment on safety issues in the tables, listings, and graphs

Monitor the extreme laboratory values and make sure they are also coded as adverse events when needed

Bias Minimization

Suggest new SMQs (standard MeDRA queries) to reduce granularity for adverse events

Beware of competing risks

Decision Making

Suggest and approve "Dear Investigator" letter

Perform "quick and dirty" risk–benefit analysis when appropriate

Contact the unmasked sponsor individual or team on safety concerns

Decision on trial continuation or termination

Use data from outside trial with caution

Conduct planned interim analysis

Request conditional power analysis when needed

In futility analysis, enforce "binding" or "nonbinding" as indicated in the protocol and DRP.

Emerging Issues

Make sure the ability of the DMC to report safety concerns are built into adaptive designs and other novel designs

Approve any change in effect size of interest taking the current safety profile into account

In basket trials make sure the DMC has the needed tumor-specific expertise

Under centralized statistical monitoring keep track of data quality metrics by site and advise the sponsor on needed improvement

In a SMART/DTS trial make sure that there is adequate safety information for the decision branches of interest

Make sure that PRO-CTCAE severity data are taken seriously

For pragmatic trials make sure all members understand that they are working on a pragmatic rather than an efficacy trial

In biosimilar trials make sure that safety differences are discussed and investigated

In event of merger or licensing make sure that patient safety is protected by independent review in the transition plan to the new sponsor

For companion diagnostics review the sensitivity, specificity, and predictive accuracy of the diagnostic and make sure that these metrics conform to scientific and industry standards

Administer the Fraud Recovery Plan when fraud is detected

For training purposes, if a DMC member resigns for a noncontroversial reason suggest replacing this person with someone who has not previously served on a DMC

References

Agresti, A. 1992. A survey of exact inference for contingency tables. *Statistical Sciences*, 7, 131–177.

Altman, D. G. 1991. *Practical Statistics for Medical Research*. London: Chapman & Hall.

Amit, O., Heiberger, R. M., and Lane, P. W. 2008. Graphical approaches to the analysis of safety data from clinical trials. *Pharmaceutical Statistics*, 7, 20–35.

Aronson, J. K. and Ferner, R. E. 2005. Clarification of terminology in drug safety. *Drug Safety*, 28, 851–870.

Arrowsmith, J. 2011a. Phase II failures: 2008–2010. *Nature Reviews Drug Discovery*, 10, 328–329.

Arrowsmith, J. 2011b. Phase III and submission failures: 2007–2010. *Nature Reviews Drug Discovery*, 10, 87.

Ashcroft, D., Li Wan Po, A., Williams, H. et al. 1999. Clinical measures of disease severity and outcome in psoriasis: A critical appraisal of their quality. *British Journal of Dermatology*, 141, 185–191.

Ball, G., Piller, L. B., and Silverman, M. H. 2011. Continuous safety monitoring for randomized controlled clinical trials with blinded treatment information. *Contemporary Clinical Trials*, 32, S1–S10.

Baron, J. A., Sandler, R. S., Bresalier, R. S. et al. 2006. A randomized trial of rofecoxib for the chemoprevention of colorectal adenomas. *Gastroenterology*, 131, 1674–1682.

Barker, A. D., Sigman, C. C., Kelloff, G. J. et al. 2009. I SPY 2: An adaptive breast cancer trial design in the setting of neoadjuvant chemotherapy. *Clinical Pharmacology and Therapeutics*, 86, 97–100.

Bathon, J. M., Martin, R. W., Fleischmann, R. M. et al. 2000. A comparison of etanercept and methotrexate in patients with early rheumatoid arthritis. *New England Journal of Medicine*, 343, 1586–1593.

Benjamini, Y. and Hochberg, Y. 1995. Controlling the false discovery rate: A practical and powerful approach to multiple testing. *Journal of the Royal Statistical Society, Series B*, 57, 289–300.

Berlin, J. A. 2008. Use of meta-analysis in drug safety assessments. Paper presented at Spring Statistical Meetings, Eastern North American Region, International Biometrics Society, Arlington, VA.

Berlin J. A., Crowe, B. J., Whalen, E. et al. 2013. Meta-analysis of clinical trial safety data in a drug development program: Answers to frequently asked questions. *Clinical Trials*, 10, 20–31.

Berry, D. A. 2005. Introduction to Bayesian methods III: Use and interpretation of Bayesian tools in design and analysis. *Clinical Trials*, 2, 295–300.

Berry, S. M. and Berry, D. A. 2004. Accounting for multiplicities in assessing drug safety: A three-level hierarchical mixture model. *Biometrics*, 60, 418–426.

Binkowitz, B. and Ibia, E. 2011. Multiregional clinical trials: An introduction from an industry perspective. *Drug Information Journal*, 45, 569–573.

Blume, J. D. 2002. Tutorial in biostatistics: Likelihood methods for measuring statistical evidence. *Statistics in Medicine*, 21, 2563–2599.

Bombardier, C., Gladman, D. D., and Urowitz, M. B. 1992. Derivation of the SLEDAI: A disease activity index for lupus patients. *Arthritis and Rheumatism*, 35, 630–640.

Bonhoeffer, J., Kohl, K., Chen, R. et al. 2002. The Brighton Collaboration addressing the need for standardized case definitions of adverse events following immunization (AEFI). *Vaccine*, 21, 298–302.

Bresalier, R. S., Sandler, R. S., Quan, H. et al. 2005. Cardiovascular events associated with rofecoxib in a colorectal adenoma chemoprevention trial. *New England Journal of Medicine*, 352, 1092–1102.

Brooks, J. C., Go, A. S., Singer, D. E. et al. 2015. Roadmap for causal inference in safety analysis. In Jiang, Q. and Xia, H. A. (eds.), *Quantitative Evaluation of Safety in Drug Development: Design, Analysis and Reporting*. Boca Raton, FL: Chapman & Hall/CRC, Chapter 10.

Brown, E. G., Wood, L., and Wood, S. 1999. The medical dictionary for regulatory activities (MedDRA). *Drug Safety*, 20, 109–117.

Bush, J. K., Dai, W. S., Dieck, G. S. et al. 2005. The art and science of risk management: A U.S. research-based industry perspective. *Drug Safety*, 28, 1–18.

Bousquet, C., Lagier, G., and Lillo-Le Louet, A. 2005. Appraisal of the MedDRA conceptual structure for describing and grouping adverse drug reactions. *Drug Safety*, 28, 19–34.

Califf, R. M., Filerman, G. L., Murray, R. K. et al. 2012. The clinical trials enterprise in the United States: A call for disruptive innovation. *Institute of Medicine Discussion Paper—IOM Forum on Drug Discovery, Development and Translation*. Washington, DC, Institute of Medicine.

Califf, R. M. and Sugarman, J. 2015. Exploring the ethical and regulatory issues in pragmatic clinical trials. *Clinical Trials*, 12, 436–441.

Caplan, A. L. 1992. Twenty years after: The legacy of the Tuskegee Syphilis Study. *Hastings Center Report*, 22, 29–32.

Carpenter, D., Zucker, E. J., and Avorn, J. 2008. Drug review deadlines and safety problems. *New England Journal of Medicine*, 358, 1354–1361.

Charney, D. S., Nemeroff, C. B., Lewis, L. et al. 2002. National Depressive and Manic-Depressive Association consensus statement on the use of placebo in clinical trials of mood disorders. *Archives of General Psychiatry*, 59, 262–270.

Chow, S.-C. 2014. *Biosimilars: Design and Analysis of Follow-on Biologics*. Boca Raton, FL: Chapman & Hall/CRC.

Chuang-Stein, C., Anderson, K., Gallo, P. et al. 2006. Sample size reestimation: A review and recommendations. *Drug Information Journal*, 40, 475–484.

Chuang-Stein, C., Entsuah, R., and Pritchett, Y. 2008. Measures for conducting comparative benefit: Risk assessment. *Drug Information Journal*, 42, 223–233.

Chuang-Stein, C. and Xia, H. A. 2013. The practice of pre-marketing safety assessment in drug development. *Journal of Biopharmaceutical Statistics*, 23, 3–25.

Cleves, M., Gould, W., Guttierrez, R. et al. 2008. *An Introduction to Survival Analysis Using Stata*, Second Ed., Boca Raton, FL: CRC Press.

Clinicaltrials.gov. 2016. *TAPUR: Testing the Use of Food and Drug Administration (FDA) Approved Drugs That Target a Specific Abnormality in a Tumor Gene in People With Advanced Stage Cancer*. https://clinicaltrials.gov/ct2/show/NCT02693535

Clopper, C. J. and Pearson, E. S. 1934. The use of confidence or fiducial limits illustrated in the case of the binomial. *Biometrika*, 26, 404–413.

Code of Federal Regulations. 2016. Protection of Human Subjects-45 CFR Part 46, http://www.ecfr.gov/cgi-bin/text-idx?tpl=/ecfrbrowse/Title45/45cfr46_main_02.tpl

Cohen, S. B., Emery, P., Greenwald, M. W. et al. 2006. Rituximab for rheumatoid arthritis refractory to anti-tumor necrosis factor therapy: Results of a multi-center, randomized, double blind placebo-controlled phase III trial evaluating primary efficacy and safety at 24 weeks. *Arthritis and Rheumatism*, 54, 2793–2806.

Cornfield, J. 1973. Remarks made at *Spring Biostatistics Meeting*. Ithaca, NY.

Council for International Organizations of Medical Sciences. 2005. *Management of Safety Information from Clinical Trials: Report of CIOMS Working Group VI*. CIOMS: Geneva Switzerland.

Council for International Organizations of Medical Sciences. 2006. *Development Safety Update Report (DSUR) Harmonizing the Format and Content for Periodic Safety Report during Clinical Trials: Report of CIOMS Working Group VII*. CIOMS: Geneva Switzerland.

Council for International Organizations of Medical Sciences. 2015. *Practical Approaches to Risk Minimisation for Medicinal Products: Report of CIOMS Working Group IX*. CIOMS: Geneva Switzerland.

Cox, D. R. 1972. Regression models and life tables (with discussion). *Journal of the Royal Statistical Society B*, 34, 187–220.

Cranney, A. and Adachi, J. D. 2005. Benefit-risk assessment of raloxifene in post-menopausal osteoporosis. *Drug Safety*, 28, 721–730.

Crowe, B. J., Xia, H. A., Berlin, J. A. et al. 2009. Recommendations for safety planning, data collection, evaluation and reporting during drug, biologic and vaccine development: A report of the safety planning, evaluation and reporting team. *Clinical Trials*, 6, 430–440.

Cui, L., Hung, M. H. J., and Wang, S. J. 1999. Modification of sample size in group sequential clinical trials. *Biometrics*, 55, 853–857.

Cytel. 2007. *StatXact 8 User Manual*. Cambridge, MA: Cytel, Inc.

Davidson, A. 2015. What Hollywood can teach us about the future of work. *New York Times Magazine*, May 5, 2015.

Davis, B. and Southworth, H. 2016. Statistical analysis of cumulative serious adverse event data from development safety reports. *Therapeutic Innovation and Regulatory Science*, 50, 188–194.

Day, R. O. and Williams, K. M. 2007. Open-label extension studies: Do they provide meaningful information on the safety of new drugs? *Drug Safety*, 30, 93–105.

Deeks, J. 1998. When can odds ratios mislead? Odds ratios should only be used in case-control studies and logistic regression analyses. *British Medical Journal*, 317, 1155–1156.

DeMets, D. L., Fleming, T. R., Rockhold, F. et al. 2004. Liability issues for data monitoring committee members. *Clinical Trials*, 1, 525–531.

DeMets, D. L., Furberg, C. D., and Friedman, L. M. 2006. *Data Monitoring in Clinical Trials: A Case Studies Approach*. New York: Springer.

DerSimonian, R. and Laird, N. 1986. Meta-analysis in clinical trials. *Controlled Clinical Trials*, 7, 177–178.

Devchand, P. R. 2008. Glitazones and the cardiovascular system. *Current Opinion in Endocrinology, Diabetes and Obesity*, 15, 188–192.

D'Agostino, R. B., Massaro, J. M., and Sullivan, L. M. 2003. Non-inferiority trials: Design concepts and issues—the encounters of academic consultants in statistics. *Statistics in Medicine*, 22, 169–186.

Dickersin, K., Olson, C. M., Rennie, D. et al. 2002. Association between time interval to publication and statistical significance: Reports of controlled trials published in JAMA. *Journal of American Medical Association*, 287, 2829–2831.

Dickersin, K. and Rennie, D. 2003. Registering clinical trials. *Journal of American Medical Association*, 290, 516–523.

Dixon, D. O., Freedman, R. S., Herson, J. et al. 2006. Guidelines for data and safety monitoring for clinical trials not requiring traditional data monitoring committees. *Clinical Trials*, 3, 314–319.

Djunaedi, E., Sommer, A., Pandji, A., Kusdiono Taylor, H. R., and the Aceh Study Group. 1988. Impact of vitamin A supplementation on xerophthalmia. A randomized controlled community trial. *Archives of Ophthalmology*, 106, 218–222.

Dragalin, V. 2006. Adaptive designs: Terminology and classification. *Drug Information Journal*, 40, 425–435.

Dueck, A. C., Mendoza, T. R., Mitchell, S. A. et al. 2015. Validity and reliability of the U.S. National Cancer Institute's Patient Reported Outcome Version of the Common Terminology Criteria for Adverse Events. *JAMA Oncology*, 1, 1051–1059.

Duke, S. P., Jiang, Q., Huang, L. et al. 2015. Safety graphics. In Jiang, Q. and Xia, H. A. (eds.), *Quantitative Evaluation of Safety in Drug Development: Design, Analysis and Reporting*. Boca Raton, FL: Chapman & Hall/CRC, Chapter 11.

Edwards, I. R. and Biriell, C. 1994. Harmonisation in pharmacovigilance. *Drug Safety*, 10, 93–102.

Ellenberg, S. S., Culbertson, R., Gillen, D. L. et al. 2015. Data monitoring committees for pragmatic clinical trials. *Clinical Trials*, 12, 530–536.

Ellenberg, S. S., Fleming, T. R., and DeMets, D. L. 2002. *Data Monitoring Committees in Clinical Trials: A Practical Perspective*. New York: John Wiley & Sons.

Ellenberg, S. S and George, S. L. 2004. Should statisticians reporting to data monitoring committees be independent of the trial sponsor and leadership? *Statistics in Medicine*, 23, 1503–1505.

Ellis, A. J., Hughes, R. D., Wendon, J. A. et al. 1996. Pilot-controlled trial of extracorporeal liver assist device in acute liver failure. *Hepatology*, 24, 1446–1451.

European Commission. 2011. Detailed guidance on the collection, verification, presentation of adverse event/reaction reports arising from clinical trials (CT-3). *Official Journal of the European Union*, 172, 1–13.

Fairweather, W. R. 1996. Integrated safety analysis: Statistical issues in the assessment of safety in clinical trials. *Drug Information Journal*, 30, 875–879.

Fanelli, D. 2009. How many scientists fabricate and falsify research? A systematic review and meta-analyses of survey data. *PLoS One*, 4, e5738, doi: 10.137/journal.pone.0005738.

Faught, E., Sachdeo, R. C., Remler, M. P. et al. 1993. Felbamate monotherapy for partial onset seizures: An active control trial. *Neurology*, 43, 688–692.

Fay, M. P., Huang, C-Y., and Twum-Danso, N. A. 2007. Monitoring rare serious adverse events from a new treatment and testing for a difference from historical controls. *Clinical Trials*, 6, 598–610.

Fleming, T. R., Hennekens, C. H., Pfeffer, M. A. et al. 2014. Enhancing trial integrity by protecting the independence of data monitoring committees in clinical trials. *Journal of Biopharmaceutical Statistics*, 24, 968–975.

FOI Services. 2008. Document search, www.foiservices.com.

Ford, J. G., Howerton, M. W., Lai, G. Y. et al. 2008. Barriers to recruiting underrepresented populations to cancer clinical trials: A systematic review. *Cancer*, 112, 228–242.

Fontanarosa, P. B., Flanagin, A., and DeAngelis, C. D. 2005. Reporting conflicts of interest, financial aspects of research and role of sponsors in funded studies. *Journal of American Medical Association*, 294, 110–111.

Frangakis, C. E. and Rubin, D. B. 2002. Principal stratification in causal inference. *Biometrics*, 58, 21–29.

Fredriksson, T. and Pettersson, U. 1978. Severe psoriasis—Oral therapy with a new retinoid. *Dermatologica*, 157, 238–244.

Friedman, L. and DeMets, D. 1981. The data monitoring committee: How it operates and why. *IRB: Ethics and Human Research*, 3, 6–8.

Friedman, M. A., Woodcock, J., Lumpkin, M. M. et al. 1999. The safety of newly approved medicines: Do recent market removals mean there is a problem? *Journal of American Medical Association*, 281, 1728–1734.

Gallo, P. 2006. Confidentiality and trial integrity issues for adaptive designs. *Drug Information Journal*, 40, 445–449.

Gallo, P. and Krams, M. 2006. PhRMA working group on adaptive designs: Introduction to the full white paper. *Drug Information Journal*, 40, 421–423.

Gart, J. 1970. Point and interval estimation of the common odds ratio in the combination of 2×2 tables with fixed marginals. *Biometrika*, 57, 471–475.

Gart, J. 1971. The comparison of proportions: A review of significance tests, confidence intervals and adjustments for stratification. *Review of the Indian Statistical Institute*, 39, 148–169.

Gelman, A., Carlin, J. B., Stern, H. S. et al. 2004. *Bayesian Data Analysis*, Second Ed., Boca Raton, FL: Chapman & Hall/CRC.

George, S. L. 2016. Research misconduct and data fraud in clinical trials: Prevalence and causal factors. *International Journal of Clinical Oncology*, 21, 15–21.

George, S. L. and Buyse, M. 2015. Data fraud in clinical trials. *Clinical Investigation*, 5, 161–173.

Gerber, D. E., Oxnard, G. R., and Govindan, R. 2015. ALCHEMIST: Bringing genomic discovery and targeted therapies to early stage lung cancer. *Clinical Pharmacology and Therapeutics*, 97, 447–450.

German Institute for Quality and Efficiency in Health Care. 2008. IQWiG Home Page http://www.iqwig.de/index.2.en.html

Geyer, C. E., Forster, J. Lindquist, D. et al. 2006. Lapatinib plus capecitabine for HER2-positive advanced breast cancer. *New England Journal of Medicine*, 355, 2733–2743.

Gibbons, R. D. and Amatya, A. K. 2016. *Statistical Methods for Drug Safety*. Boca Raton, FL: Chapman and Hall/CRC.

Glaser, A. 2002. A set of quality criteria for statistical programming. *Drug Information Journal*, 36, 565–570.

Glass, G. V. 1976. Primary, secondary and meta-analysis of research. *Educational Researcher*, 5, 3–8.

Goldman, S. A. 2002. Adverse event reporting and standard medical terminologies: Strengths and limitations. *Drug Information Journal*, 36, 439–444.

Gorelik, P. B., Harris, Y., Burnett, B. et al. 1998. The recruitment triangle: Reasons why African Americans enroll, refuse to enroll or voluntarily withdraw from a clinical trial. *Journal of the National Medical Association*, 90, 141–145.

Gould, A. L. 2013. Personal communication.

Gould, A. L. 2015. Safety graphics. In Gould, A. L. (ed.), *Statistical Methods for Evaluating Safety in Medical Product Development*. Chichester, West Sussex: John Wiley & Sons, Ltd., Chapter 2.

Gould, A. L. and Wang, W. 2016. Monitoring potential adverse event rate differences using data from blinded trials: The canary in the coal mine. *Statistics in Medicine*. DOI: 10.1002/sim.7129.

Gray, R. J. 1988. A class of k-sample tests for comparing the cumulative incidence of a competing risk. *Annals of Statistics*, 16, 1141–1154.

Grunkenmeier, G. L., Jin, R., and Starr, A. 2006. Prosthetic heart valves: Objective performance criteria vs. randomized clinical trial. *Annals of Thoracic Surgery*, 82, 776–780.

Grunkenmeier, G. L., Johnson, D. M., and Naftel, D. C. 1994. Sample size requirements for evaluating heart valves with constant risk events. *The Journal of Heart Valve Disease*, 3, 53–58.

Guo, J. J., Pandey, S., Doyle, J. et al. 2010. A review of quantitative risk–benefit methodologies for assessing drug safety and efficacy—Report of the ISPOR risk–benefit management working group. *Value Health*, 13, 657–666.

Haas, J. F. 2004. A problem-oriented approach to safety issues in drug development and beyond. *Drug Safety*, 27, 555–567.

Habermann, T. M., Weller, E. A., Morrison, V. A. et al. 2006. Rituximab–CHOP versus CHOP alone or with maintenance rituximab in older patients with diffuse large B-cell lymphoma. *Journal of Clinical Oncology*, 24, 3121–3127.

Hamilton, M. 1960. A rating scale for depression. *Journal of Neurology, Neurosurgery and Psychiatry*, 23, 56–62.

Hammad, T. A., Neyarapally, G. A., Pinhiero, S. P. et al. 2013. Reporting of meta-analyses of randomized controlled trials with a focus on drug safety: An empirical assessment. *Clinical Trials*, 10, 389–397.

Harris, G. 2007. FDA issues strictest warning on diabetes drugs. *New York Times*, June 7, 2007.

Harvey, S., Harrison, D. A., Singer, M. et al. 2005. Assessment of the clinical effectiveness of pulmonary artery catheters in management of patients in intensive care (PAC-Man): A randomised controlled trial. *Lancet*, 366, 472–477.

Havel, R. J., Hunninghake, D. B., Illingworth, D. R. et al. 1987. Lovastatin (mevinolin) in the treatment of heterozygous familial hypercholesterolemia—A multicenter study. *Annals of Internal Medicine*, 107, 609–615.

Haybittle, J. L. 1971. Repeated assessment of results in clinical trials of cancer treatment. *British Journal of Radiology*, 44, 793–797.

Heiat, A., Gross, C. P., and Krumholz, H. M. 2002. Representation of the elderly, women and minorities in heart failure trials. *Archives of Internal Medicine*, 162(15), doi 10.1001/archinte162.15.1682.

Hemmings, R. and Day, S. 2004. Regulatory perspectives on data safety monitoring boards: Protecting the integrity of data. *Drug Safety*, 27, 1–6.

Herbst, R. S., Gandara, D. R., Hirsch, F. R. et al. 2015. Lung master protocol (Lung-MAP): A biomarker-driven protocol for accelerating development of therapies for squamous cell lung cancer. *Clinical Cancer Research*, 21, 1514–1524.

Herson, J. 1993. Data monitoring boards in the pharmaceutical industry. *Statistics in Medicine*, 12, 555–561.

Herson, J. 2008. Coordinating data monitoring committees and adaptive clinical trial designs. *Drug Information Journal*, 42, 297–301.

Herson, J. 2015a. Safety monitoring. In Gould, A. L. (ed.), *Statistical Methods for Evaluating Safety in Medical Product Development*. Chichester, West Sussex: John Wiley & Sons, Ltd., Chapter 11.

Herson, J. 2015b. Global drug safety: 2030. *World Future Review*, 6, 441–447.

Herson, J. 2016. Strategies for dealing with fraud in clinical trials. *International Journal of Clinical Oncology*, 21, 23–27.

Herson, J., Buyse, M., and Wittes, J. T. 2012. On stopping a randomized clinical trial for futility. In Harrington, D. (ed.), *Designs for Clinical Trials: Perspectives on Current Issues*. New York: Springer, Chapter 5.

Herson, J., Ognibene, F. P., Peura, D. A. et al. 1992. The role of an independent data monitoring board in a clinical trial sponsored by a pharmaceutical firm. *Journal of Clinical Research and Pharmacoepidemiology*, 6, 285–292

Hibberd, P. L. and Weiner, D. L. 2004. Monitoring participant safety in phase I and II interventional trials: Options and controversies. *Journal of Investigative Medicine*, 52, 446–452.

Hollander, M. and Wolfe, D. A. 1999. *Nonparametric Statistical Methods*, Second Ed., New York: John Wiley.

Hosmer, D. W. and Lemeshow, S. 2000. *Applied Logistic Regression*. New York: Wiley.

Ibrahim, J. G., Chen, M. H., Xia, H. A. et al. 2012. Bayesian meta-experimental design: Evaluating cardiovascular risk in new antidiabetic therapies to treat type 2 diabetes. *Biometrics*, 68, 578–576.

International Conference on Harmonisation. 1994. *E2A: Clinical Safety Data Management: Definitions and Standards for Expedited Reporting.* Geneva, Switzerland: ICH.

International Conference on Harmonisation. 1995. *E3: Structure and Content of Clinical Study Reports.* Geneva, Switzerland: ICH.

International Conference on Harmonisation. 1996. *E6: Guideline for Good Clinical Practice.* Geneva, Switzerland: ICH.

International Conference on Harmonisation. 1998. *E9: Statistical Principles for Clinical Trials.* Geneva, Switzerland: ICH.

International Conference on Harmonisation. 2007. *MedDRA Data Retrieval and Presentation: Points to Consider.* Geneva, Switzerland: ICH.

International Conference on Harmonisation. 2010. *Development Safety Update Report-E2F.* Geneva, Switzerland: ICH.

International Conference on Harmonisation. 2012. *Periodic Benefit-Risk Evaluation Report (PBRER)—E2C(R2).* Geneva, Switzerland: ICH.

Ioannidis, J. P. A., Evans, S. J. W., Getzsche, P. C. et al. 2004. Better reporting of harms in randomized trials: An extension of the CONSORT statement. *Annals of Internal Medicine*, 141, 781–788.

Ioannidis, J. P. A. and Lau, J. 2002. Improving safety reporting from randomized trials. *Drug Safety*, 25, 77–84.

Ioannidis, J. P. A., Mulrow, C. D., and Goodman, S. N. 2006. Adverse events: The more you search, the more you find (editorial). *Annals of Internal Medicine*, 144, 298–300.

Johann-Liang, R., James, A. N., Behr, V. L. et al. 2005. Reporting of deaths during preapproval clinical trials for advanced HIV-infected populations. *Drug Safety*, 28, 559–564.

Kahn, J. 2006. A nation of guinea pigs. *Wired*, 14.03, 277–283.

Kaplan, E. L. and Meier, P. 1958. Nonparametric estimation from incomplete observations. *Journal of the American Statistical Association*, 53, 457–480.

Ke, C., Jiang, Q., and Snapinn, S. 2015. Risk–benefit assessment approaches. In Jiang, Q. and Xia, H. A. (eds.), *Quantitative Evaluation of Safety in Drug Development: Design, Analysis and Reporting.* Boca Raton, FL: Chapman & Hall/CRC, Chapter 15.

Kirkwood, A., Cox, T., and Hackshaw, A. 2013. Application of methods for central statistical monitoring in clinical trials. *Clinical Trials*, 10, 783–806.

Klein, J. P., Logan, B., Harhoff, M. et al. 2007. Analyzing survival curves at a fixed point in time. *Statistics in Medicine*, 26, 4505–4519.

Kubler, J., Vonk, R., Belmel, S. et al. 2005. Adverse event analysis and MedDRA: Business as usual or challenge? *Drug Information Journal*, 39, 63–72.

Lachin, J. M. 2004. Conflicts of interest in data monitoring of industry versus publicly financed clinical trials. *Statistics in Medicine*, 23, 1519–1521.

Lan, K. and DeMets, D. 1983. Discrete sequential boundaries for clinical trials. *Biometrika*, 70, 659–663.

Lan, K. K. G., Hu, P., and Proschan, M. A. 2009. A conditional power approach to the evaluation of predictive power. Accepted, *Statistics in Biopharmaceutical Research*, 1, 131–136.

Lasser, K. E., Allen, P. D., Woolhandler, S. J. et al. 2002. Timing of new black box warnings and withdrawals for prescription medications. *Journal of American Medical Association*, 287, 2215–2220.

Lassere, M. N. D., Johnson, K. P., Boers, M. et al. 2005. Standardized assessment of adverse events in rheumatology clinical trials: Summary of the OMERACT 7 drug safety module update. *Journal of Rheumatology*, 32, 2037–2041.

Laupacis, A., Sackett, D. L., and Roberts, R. S. 1988. An assessment of clinically useful measures of the consequences of treatment. *New England Journal of Medicine*, 318, 1728–1733.

Lavori, P. W. and Dawson, R. 2014. Introduction to dynamic treatment strategies and sequential multiple assignment randomization. *Clinical Trials*, 11, 393–399.

Lechleiter, J. H. 2014. Closing the diversity gap in clinical trials. *Forbes*, April 9, 2014.

Lee, Y. H., Ji, J. D., and Song, G. G. 2007. Adjusted indirect comparison of celecoxib verses rofecoxib on cardiovascular risk. *Pharmacology International*, 27, 477–482.

Lenz, H.-J., Van Cutsem, E., Khambata-Ford, S. et al. 2006. Multicenter phase II and translational study of cetuximab in metastatic colorectal carcinoma refractory to irinotecan, oxaliplatin and fluoropyrimidines. *Journal of Clinical Oncology*, 24, 4914–4921.

Levitan, B. S., Andrews, E. B., Gilsenan, A. et al. 2011. Application of the BRAT framework to case studies: Observations and insights. *Clinical Pharmacology and Therapeutics*, 89, 217–224.

Lewis, P. A., O'Sullivan, M. M., and Rumfield, W. R. 1988. Significant changes in Ritchie scores. *Rheumatology*, 27, 32–36.

Liberati, A., Altman D. G., Tetzlaff, J. et al. 2009. The PRISMA statement for reporting systematic reviews and meta-analyses of studies that evaluate health care interventions: Explanation and elaboration. *Annals of Internal Medicine*, 15, W65–W94.

Lin, Y.-L, Chern, H.-D., and Chu, M.-L. 2003. Hepatotoxicity in the review of clinical safety data. *Drug Information Journal*, 37, 155–158.

Lipid Research Clinics Program. 1984a. The Lipid Research Clinics Coronary Prevention Trial results I. *Journal of the American Medical Association*, 251, 351–364.

Lipid Research Clinics Program. 1984b. The Lipid Research Clinics Coronary Prevention Trial results II. *Journal of the American Medical Association*, 251, 365–374.

Luan, J. J., Muni, R., and Hung, H. M. J. 2016. Comparison of treatment effects between U.S. and non-U.S. study sites in multiregional Alzheimer's disease clinical trials. *Therapeutic Innovation and Regulatory Science*, 50, 66–73.

Lurie, P. and Sasich, L. D. 1999. Safety of FDA-approved drugs. *Journal of American Medical Association*, 282, 2297–2298.

Magin, P. and Smith, W. 2005. Isotretinoin, depression and suicide: A review of the evidence. *British Journal of General Practice*, 55, 134–138.

Martin, L. F., Booth, F. V., Karlstadt, R. G. et al. 1993. Continuous intravenous cimetidine decreased stress-related upper gastrointestinal hemorrhage without promoting pneumonia. *Critical Care Medicine*, 21, 19–30.

Mayer, R. J., Van Cutsem, E., Falcone, A. et al. 2015. Randomized trial of TAS-102 for refractory metastatic colorectal cancer. *New England Journal of Medicine*, 372, 1909–1919.

McNeill, C. 2015. NCI-MATCH launch highlights new trial design in precision medicine era. *Journal of the National Cancer Institute*, 107, djv193, doi: 10.1093/jnci/djv193.

MedCalc. 2016a. Relative risk calculator. https://www.medcalc.org/calc/relative_risk.php

MedCalc. 2016b. Odds ratio calculator. https://www.medcalc.org/calc/odds_ratio.php.

MedDRA. 2013. MedDRA Maintenance Support and Services Organization. Introductory Guide for Stanardized MedDRA Queries, Version 16.0.

MedDRA. 2016. MedDRA Maintenance Support and Services Organization. www.meddra.org.

Mehrotra, D. V. and Adewale, A. J. 2012. Flagging clinical adverse event experiences: Reducing false discoveries without materially compromising power for detecting true signals. *Statistics in Medicine*, 31, 556–683.

Mehrotra, D. V. and Heyse, J. 2004. Use of the false discovery rate for evaluating clinical safety data. *Statistical Methods in Medical Research*, 13, 227–238.

Melzack, R. and Torgerson, W. S. 1971. On the language of pain. *Anesthesiology*, 34, 50–59.

MERIT-HF Study Group. 1999. Effect of metropolol CR/XL in chronic heart failure. *Lancet*, 353, 2001–2007.

Meyboom, R. H. B., Lindquist, M., and Egberts, A. C. G. 2000. An ABC of drug-related problems. *Drug Safety*, 22, 414–423.

Mikuls, T. R. and Moreland, L. W. 2003. Benefit-risk assessment of infliximab in the treatment of rheumatoid arthritis. *Drug Safety*, 26, 23–32.

Mundy, A. 2008. Drugs' links to suicide risk draw concerns. *Wall Street Journal* http://w.wsj.com/articles/SB121556144610237551

Murthy, V. H., Krumholz, H. M., and Gross, C. P. 2004. Participation in cancer clinical trials: Race, sex and age-based disparities. *Journal of American Medical Association*, 291, 2720–2726.

Ng, H. K. T. and Tang, M.-L. 2005. Testing the equality of two Poisson means using the rate ratio. *Statistics in Medicine*, 24, 955–965.

Nissen, S. E. and Wolski, K. 2007. Effect of rosiglitazone on the risk of myocardioal infarction and death from cardiovascular causes. *New England Journal of Medicine*, 356, 2457–2471.

Nissen, S. E., Wolski, K., and Topol, E. J. 2005. Effect of muraglitazar on death and major adverse cardiovascular events in patients with type 2 diabetes mellitus. *Journal of American Medical Association*, 294, 2581–2586.

O'Brien, P. C. and Fleming, T. R. 1979. A multiple testing procedure for clinical trials. *Biometrics*, 35, 549–556.

O'Neill, R. 2007. *Remarks Made at Drug Information Association/FDA Statistics Forum.* Bethesda, MD.

Patnaik, A., Kang, S. P., Rasco, D. et al. 2015. Phase I study of prembrolizumab in patients with advanced solid tumors. *Clinical Cancer Research*, 21, 4286–4293.

Pharmadhoc. 2016. NCI CTC at www.pharmadhoc.com.

Piantadosi, S. 2005. *Clinical Trials: A Methodological Perspective*, Second Ed., Hobokon, NJ: John Wiley & Sons.

Piccart-Gebhart, M., Holmes, E., Baselga, J. et al. 2016. Adjuvant lapatinib and trastuzumab for early human epidermal growth factor receptor 2—Positive breast cancer results from the randomized phase III adjuvant lapatinib and/or trastuzumab treatment optimization trial (ALTTO). *Journal of Clinical Oncology*, 34, 1034–1042.

Pintilie, M. 2006. *Competing Risks: A Practical Perspective.* West Sussex, England: John Wiley & Sons.

Platonov, P. 2003. Clinical trials in Russia and Eastern Europe: Recruitment and quality. *International Journal of Clinical Pharmacology and Therapeutics*, 41, 277–280.

Pocock, S. J. 1983. *Clinical Trials: A Practical Approach.* New York: John Wiley & Sons.

Pounds, S. and Cheng, C. 2006. Robust estimation of the false discovery rate. *Bioinformatics*, 22, 1979–1987.

Powell, J. H., Fleming, Y., and Walker-McGill, C. L. 2008. The Project IMPACT experience to date: Increasing minority participation and awareness of clinical trials. *Journal of the National Medical Association*, 100, 178–187.

Proschan, M. A., Lan, K. K. G., and Wittes, J. T. 2006. *Statistical Monitoring of Clinical Trials: A Unified Approach.* New York: Springer.

Quereshi, Z. P., Seoane-Vazquez, E., Rodriquez-Monguio, R. et al. 2011. Market withdrawal of new molecular entities approved in the United States from 1980–2009. *Pharmacoepidemiology and Drug Safety*, 20, 772–777.

Rochester, G. 2008. *Remarks Made at Spring Statistical Meetings, Eastern North American Region.* Arlington, VA: International Biometrics Society.

Rohde, C. A. 2014. *Introductory Statistical Inference with the Likelihood Function.* New York: Springer.

Rosenbaum, P. R. and Rubin, D. B. 1983. The central role of the propensity score in observational studies for causal effects. *Biometrika*, 70, 41–55.

Rosner, B. 2006. *Fundamentals of Biostatistics*, Sixth Ed., Pacific Grove, CA: Duxbury Press.

Royall, R. M. 1997. *Statistical Evidence: A Likelihood Paradigm.* London: Chapman & Hall.

Royall, R. M. 2000. On the probability of observing misleading statistical evidence (with discussion). *Journal of the American Statistical Association*, 95, 760–767.

Rush, A. J., Marangell, L. B., Sackheim, H. A. et al. 2005. Vagus nerve stimulation for treatment-resistant depression: A randomized controlled acute phase trial. *Biological Psychiatry*, 58, 347–354.

Ryan, P., Madigan, D., and Schuemie, M. J. 2015. Emerging role of observational healthcare data in pharmacovigilence. In Jiang, Q. and Xia, H. A. (eds.), *Quantitative Evaluation of Safety in Drug Development: Design, Analysis and Reporting.* Boca Raton, FL: Chapman & Hall/CRC, Chapter 9.

Sackett, D. L. 1979. Bias in analytic research. *Journal of Chronic Disease*, 32, 51–63.

SAS Institute. 2008. SAS Online Doc 9.13, SAS/STAT User's Guide, Introduction to Survival Analysis Procedures, http://support.sas.com/onlinedoc/913/docMainpage.jsp

Schactman, M. and Wittes, J. 2015. Why a DMC safety report differs from a safety section written at the end of the trial. In Jiang, Q. and Xia, H. A. (eds.), *Quantitative Evaluation of Safety in Drug Development: Design, Analysis and Reporting.* Boca Raton, FL: Chapman & Hall/CRC, Chapter 5.

Scheiner, L. B. 1997. Learning vs. confirming in clinical drug development. *Clinical Pharmacology and Therapeutics*, 61, 275–291.

Schemper, M. and Smith, T. L. 1996. A note on quantifying follow-up in studies of failure time. *Controlled Clinical Trials*, 17, 343–346.

Schilsky, R. L., Michels, D. K., and Kearbey, A. H. 2014. Building a rapid learning health care system for oncology: The regulatory framework of CancerLinq. *Journal of Clinical Oncology*, 32, 2373–2379.

Schneider, M. G., Swearingen, C. J., Schulman, L. et al. 2009. Minority enrollment in Parkinson's disease clinical trials. *Parkinsonism and Related Disorders*, 15, 258–262.

Schnell, P. and Ball, G. 2016. A Bayesian method for clinical trial safety monitoring with blinded data. *Therapeutic Innovation and Regulatory Science*, doi: 10.1177/2168479016656702.

Schoenfeld, P. 1999. Gastrointestinal safety profile of meloxicam: A meta-analysis and systematic review of randomized controlled trials. *American Journal of Medicine*, 107, 48S–54S.

Schuchman, M. 2007. Approving the vagus-nerve stimulator for depression. *New England Journal of Medicine*, 356, 1604–1607.

Shah, A., Stewart, A. K., Kolacevski, A. et al. 2016. Building a rapid learning health care system for oncology: Why CancarLinq collects identifiable health information to achieve its vision. *Journal of Clinical Oncology*, 34, 756–763.

Siegel, J. P., O'Neil, R. T., Temple, R. et al. 2004. Independence of the statistician who analyses unblinded data. *Statistics in Medicine*, 23, 1527–1529.

Siu, L. L. and Rowinsky, E. K. 1998. A risk–benefit assessment of irinotecan in solid tumors. *Drug Safety*, 18, 395–417.

Snapinn, S., Cook, T., Shapiro, D. et al. 2004. The role of the unblinded sponsor statistician. *Statistics in Medicine*, 23, 1531–1533.

Southworth, H. and O'Connell, M. 2009. Data mining and statistically guided clinical review of adverse event data in clinical trials. *Journal of Biopharmaceutical Statistics*, 19, 803–817.

Strampel, W., Emkey, R., and Civitelli, R. 2007. Safety considerations with bisphosphonates for the treatment of osteoporosis. *Drug Safety*, 30, 755–763.

Sydes, M. R., Spiegelhalter, D. J., Altman, D. G. et al. 2004. Systematic qualitative review of the literature on data monitoring committees for randomized controlled trials. *Clinical Trials*, 1, 60–79.

Temple, R. 2003. Personal communication.

Thijs, L., Celis, H., Kiowski, W. et al. 1995. Double-blind comparison of antihypertensive treatment with ramipril and piretanide, given alone or in combination. *Journal of Cardiovascular Pharmacology*, 26, 33–38.

Timmermans, C., Doffague, E., Venet, D. et al. 2016. Statistical monitoring of data quality and consistency in the stomach cancer adjuvant multi-institutional group trial. *Gastric Cancer*, 19, 24–30.

Timmermans, C., Venet, D., and Burzykowski, T. 2016. Data-driven risk identification in phase III clinical trials using centralized statistical monitoring. *International Journal of Clinical Oncology*, 21, 38–45.

Topol, E. 2012. *The Creative Destruction of Medicine: How the Digital Revolution Will Create Better Health Care*. New York: Basic Books.

Tsuburaya, A., Yoshida, K., Kobayashi, M. et al. 2014. Sequential paclitaxel followed by tegafur and uracil (UFT) or S-1 versus UFT or S-1 monotherapy as adjuvant chemotherapy for T4a/b gastric cancer (SAMIT): A phase III factorial randomized controlled trial. *Lancet Oncology*, 15, 886–893.

U.K. National Health Service. 2008. National Institute for Health and Clinical Excellence, http://www.nice.org.uk/

U.S. Food and Drug Administration. 1997. *Expedited Safety Reporting Requirements for Human Drug and Biological Products*, http://www.fda.gov/ScienceResearch/SpecialTopics/RunningClinicalTrials/ucm120262.htm

U.S. Food and Drug Administration. 2002. Safety-Based Drug Withdrawals (1997–2001), http://www.fda.gov/Safety/Recalls/ArchiveRecalls/default.htm

U.S. Food and Drug Administration. 2004a. *Innovation Stagnation: Challenge and Opportunity on the Critical Path to New Medical Products*, http://www.fda.gov/oc/initiatives/criticalpath/whitepaper.html

U.S. Food and Drug Administration. 2004b. Guidance for Industry: Premarketing Risk Assessment.

U.S. Food and Drug Administration. 2005. Guidance for Industry: Development and Use of Risk Minimization Action Plans.

U.S. Food and Drug Administration. 2006. Guidance for Clinical Trial Sponsors: Establishment and Operation of Clinical Trial Data Monitoring Committees, http://www.fda.gov/RegulatoryInformation/Guidances/ucm127069.htm

U.S. Food and Drug Administration. 2008a. *MedWatch Home Page* http://www.fda.gov/medwatch/

U.S. Food and Drug Administration. 2008b. Guidance for Industry: Diabetes Mellitus—Evaluating Cardiovascular Risk in New Antidiabetic Therapies to Treat Type 2 Diabetes.

U.S. Food and Drug Administration. 2008c. https://www.accessdata.fda.gov/scripts/cder/drugsatfda/

U.S. Food and Drug Administration. 2010. *The Sentinel Initiative: A National Strategy for Monitoring Medical Product Safety*. http://www.fda.gov/Safety/FDAsSentinelInitiative/ucm089474.htm

U.S. Food and Drug Administration. 2012. Guidance for Industry and Investigators. Safety Reports Required for INDs and BA/BE Studies.

U.S. Food and Drug Administration. 2013. Guidance for Industry. Oversight of Clinical Investigations. A Risk-Based Approach to Monitoring.

U.S. Food and Drug Administration. 2014. *In Vitro* Companion Diagnostic Devices: Guidance for Industry and Food and Drug Administration Staff.

U.S. Food and Drug Administration. 2015a. Safety Assessment for IND Safety Reporting—Draft Guidance for Industry.

U.S. Food and Drug Administration. 2015b. *Risk Evaluation and Mitigation Strategies: Modifications and Revisions*. Guidance for Industry.

U.S. Food and Drug Administration. 2015c. *A Brief Overview of Risk Evaluation and Mitigation Strategies*. http://www.fda.gov/downloads/AboutFDA/Transparency/Basics/UCM328784.pdf

U.S. Food and Drug Administration. 2016. Guidance for Industry: Determining the Extent of Safety Data Collection Needed in Late-Stage Premarket and Postapproval Clinical Investigations.

U.S. National Cancer Institute. 2006. Cancer Therapy Evaluation Program, *Common Terminology Criteria for Adverse Events v3.0 (CTCAE)*, https://ctep.cancer.gov/protocolDevelopment/electronic_applications/docs/ctcaev3.pdf

U.S. National Cancer Institute. 2013. Patient Reported Outcomes Version of the Common Terminology Criteria for Adverse Events. http://deainfo.nci.nih.gov/advisory/ctac/archive/1113/PRO-CTCAE.pdf

U.S. National Cancer Institute. 2016. Patient Reported Outcomes Version of the Common Terminology Criteria for Adverse Events. http://healthcaredelivery.cancer.gov/pro-ctcae/

U.S. National Institute of Allergy and Infectious Disease. 2007. Division of Microbiology and Infectious Diseases, *Adult Toxicity Table*, https://www.niaid.nih.gov/LabsAndResources/resources/DMIDClinRsrch/Documents/dmidadulttox.pdf

U.S. National Institutes of Health. 1998. NIH policy for data and safety monitoring, http://grants.nih.gov/grants/guide/notice-files/not98-084.html

U.S. National Institutes of Health. 1999. Guidance on reporting adverse events to Institutional Review Boards for NIH multicenter trials, http://grants.nih.gov/grants/guide/notice-files/not99-107.html

U.S. National Institutes of Health. 2000. Further guidance on data and safety monitoring for phase I and II trials, http://grants.nih.gov/grants/guide/notice-files/NOT-OD-00-038.html

U.S. Supreme Court. 1964. *Jacobellis v. Ohio*, 378 U.S. 184, http://www.aegis.com/law/SCt/Decisions/1964/378US184.html

van Oers, N. H. J., Klasa, R., Marcus, R. E. et al. 2006. Rituximab maintenance improves clinical outcome of relapse resistant follicular non-Hodgkins lymphoma in patients both with and without rituximab during induction: Results of a prospective randomized phase III intergroup trial. *Blood*, 108, 3295–3301.

Venet, D., Doffagne, E., Burzykowski, T. et al. 2012. A statistical approach to central monitoring of data quality in clinical trials. *Clinical Trials*, 9, 705–713.

Venulet, J. and Bankowski, Z. 1998. Harmonizing adverse drug reaction terminology: The role of the Council for International Organizations of Medical Sciences. *Drug Safety*, 19, 165–172.

Wacker, B., Nagrani, T., Weinberg, J. et al. 2007. Correlation between development of rash and efficacy in patients treated with the epidermal growth factor receptor tyrosine kinase inhibitor erlotinib in two large phase III studies. *Clinical Cancer Research*, 13, 3913–3921.

Wallentin, L., Becker, R. C., Budaj, A. et al. for the PLATO Investigators. 2009. Ticagrelor versus clopidogrel in patients with acute coronary syndromes. *New England Journal of Medicine*, 361, 1045–1057.

Weihrauch, T. R. and Kubler, J. 2002. Integrated summaries and meta-analyses in clinical drug development. *Drug Information Journal*, 36, 127–133.

Wernicke, J. F., Faries, D., Milton, D. et al. 2005. Detecting treatment-emergent adverse events in clinical trials—A comparison of spontaneously reported and solicited collection methods. *Drug Safety*, 28, 1057–1063.

Wernicke, J., Lledo, A., and Raskin, J. 2007. An evaluation of the cardiovascular safety profile of duloxetine: Findings from 42 placebo-controlled studies. *Drug Safety*, 30, 437–455.

White, C. A. 1998. A preliminary assessment of the impact of MedDRA on adverse event reports and product labeling. *Drug Information Journal*, 32, 347–362.

Whitehead, A. 2002. *Meta-Analysis of Controlled Clinical Trials*. West Sussex, England: John Wiley & Sons.

Wilson, J. F., Weale, M. F., Smith, A. C. et al. 2001. Population genetics structures of variable drug response. *Nature Genetics*, 29, 265–269.

Wittes, J., Barrett-Connor, E., Braunwald, E. et al. 2007. Monitoring the randomized trials of the Women's Health Initiative: The experience of the data and safety monitoring board. *Clinical Trials*, 4, 218–234.

Wittes, J., Crowe, B., Chuang-Stein, C. et al. 2015. The FDAs final rule on expedited safety reporting: Statistical considerations. *Statistics in Biopharmaceutical Research*, 7, 174–190.

Woodin, K. E. and Schneider, J. C. 2003. *The CRAs Guide to Monitoring Clinical Research*. Boston: Thompson Center Watch.

Writing Group for the Women's Health Initiative Investigators. 2002. Risks and benefits of estrogen plus progestin in health postmenopausal women—Principal results from the Women's Health Initiative randomized controlled trial. *Journal of American Medical Association*, 288, 321–333.

Wysowski, D. K. and Swartz, L. 2005. Adverse drug event surveillance and drug withdrawals in the United States, 1969–2002. *Archives of Internal Medicine*, 165, 1363–1369.

Xia, H. A., Crowe, B. J., Schriver, R. C. et al. 2011. Planning and core analyses for periodic aggregate safety data reviews. *Clinical Trials*, 8, 175–182.

Xia, H.A. and Jiang, Q. 2014. Statistical evaluation of drug safety data. *Therapeutic Innovation & Regulatory Science*, 48, 109–120.

Xia, H. A., Ma, H., and Carlin, B. P. 2011. Bayesian hierarchical modeling for detecting safety signals in clinical trials. *Journal of Biopharmaceutical Statistics*, 21, 1006–1029.

Ziemssen, T., Neuhaus, O., and Hohlfield, R. 2001 Risk–benefit assessment of glatiramer acetate in multiple sclerosis. *Drug Safety*, 24, 979–990.

Zink, R. C., Wolfinger, R. D., and Mann, G. 2013. Summarizing incidence of adverse events using volcano plots and time intervals. *Clinical Trials*, 10, 398–406.

Zuckerman, J., van de Schalie, B., and Cahill, K. 2015. Developing training for data safety monitoring board members: A National Institute for Allergic and Infectious Diseases case study. *Clinical Trials*, 12, 688–691.

Index

Printed in the United States
by Baker & Taylor Publisher Services